PRAISE FOR DISRUPTIVE BEHAVIOR

Disruptive Behavior, by four Stanford University child and adolescent psychiatrists, is a treasure trove of useful information about these difficult conditions. A real plus is the engaging, first person writing style that holds the reader's interest far more than most texts. As a forensic child and adolescent psychiatrist, I often see how serious disruptive behaviors can bring youth into contact with the juvenile justice system. This volume's in-depth exploration of those behaviors will help the reader immensely in assessing delinquents' needs for treatment, formulating clear treatment plans for youth both in and out of detention, and guiding towards much needed improvements in the systems of care for troubled youth. An extremely valuable resource!

—**Peter Ash, MD**
Professor and Director
Psychiatry and Law Service
Emory University

One in seven children are diagnosed with a childhood disruptive behavior disorder and we are only now starting to realize the enormous social, financial and legal implications associated with these diagnoses. Professor Hans Steiner is one of the leading experts on childhood disruptive behavior disorders. In this highly readable book, he and his co-authors impressively and definitively cover the field. They provide comprehensive reviews of the historical emergence of the recognition that many individuals with atypically aggressive behavior show these problems because of a psychiatric condition as well as definitive chapters on the taxonomy, epidemiology, etiology, treatment and implications for the justice system. Each chapter is penetrating in its analysis and, critically, provides not only a context for the current problems in the specific area but also clear guidelines as to how these problems can be ameliorated. As such, this definitive work will serve as a pre-eminent guide for graduate students, clinicians and researchers interested in the area alike.

—**Dr. R.J.R. Blair**
Director, Center of Neurobehavioral Research
Boys Town National Research Hospital
2017 Visiting Professor,
Program in Psychiatry & The Law
Stanford University, School, of Medicine

'Disruptive Behavior: Development, Psychopathology, Crime and Treatment" by Steiner, Daniels, Kelly, and Stadler struck me, after having read so many of these books, apart from its up-to-dateness, by its positive and inspiring tone used while reviewing the literature, and by its stimulating, hope giving tone for practitioners. This textbook addresses therapeutic and services issues on a science based level, but so accessible that every professional will learn from it and will be able to apply it in daily assessment and treatment activities, in clinical settings but in forensic contexts as well. This superb book will certainly be the standard reference for the specialty for years to come! It provides excellent steps in right directions, like speaking of 'DBD-spectrum disorders'. I would stress the importance of this textbook by citing this exemplary sentence: *Fortunately, there is also evidence that early intervention with such high-CU children holds the promise of restoring their developmental progress, when using a multimodal treatment package with a high level of parental involvement, focused on the creation of a warm supportive parent child relationship which facilitates emotional learning.*

—**Theo Doreleijers MD PhD**
Em. prof. of child and adolescent psychiatry,
VU Univ. medical centre, Amsterdam
Em. prof. of forensic psychiatry, Law Faculty, Leiden University
Honorary president of Europ. Assoc. for forensic ch&adol
psychiatry and psychology EFCAP
Best VU University Teacher Award 2012
Societal Impact Research Award VU University 2010a

—**Arne Popma MD PhD,** child and adolescent psychiatrist
Head of the dpt. of child and adolescent psychiatry,
VU University medical centre Amsterdam
Prof. of forensic psychiatry, Law Faculty, Leiden University
Chairman of EFCAP Netherlands

In an era of constraining resources for health care, very few health issues have the the potential to improve the lives of the children and families we treat and simultaneously reduce costs for the health, judicial and social welfare systems. This book stands apart from others in the field by laying out a pragmatic framework for addressing childhood aggression and disruptive behaviors. While clinicians and academics will find much insight in this book, many parents might likewise benefit from a nuanced view of the problems they face with their children. Aggression in childhood is normal, but unchecked it results in children with behavioral problems, families with stress, and societies with expensive jails and health care systems. Read this book and learn the way forward for us to change this trajectory.

—**Niranjan S. Karnik, MD, PhD** | Cynthia Oudejans Harris Professor
Vice Chair for Innovation | Department of Psychiatry
Medical Director | Road Home Program: Center for
Veterans & their Families
Director | Section of Population Behavioral Health |
Department of Psychiatry

Few constructs, if any, have led to similar plethora of research and debate across policy and practice as youth aggression, antisocial or disruptive behavior. The reasons are related to the high prevalence, complexity, comorbidity, heterogeneity and multi-factorial etiology; in parallel with the resulting impact, impairment, inter-agency involvement, and high service and societal costs. The literature stems for a range of scientific fields, which reflects children and youth's multiple needs, hence appropriate interventions. The wider connotations of criminality and its causes often divide policy in the philosophy underpinning juvenile systems across the world.

The authors, with their strong track record and all-encompassing analytic, thoughtful and succinct writing style succeed in integrating the evidence behind such a complex topic. As implications for policy, service, practice and services from different sectors are best understood in their totality, this is the major contribution of this excellent text.

—**Panos Vostanis**
Professor of Child Mental Health, University of Leicester
Visiting Professor, University College London
8th December 2016

DISRUPTIVE BEHAVIOR

DEVELOPMENT, PSYCHOPATHOLOGY, CRIME, AND TREATMENT

HANS STEINER, MD
Professor Emeritus (Active) of Psychiatry and Human Development
Director, Program in Psychiatry and the Law
Stanford University School of Medicine

WHITNEY DANIELS, MD
Clinical Instructor of Psychiatry and Behavioral Sciences
Division of Child and Adolescent Psychiatry
Stanford University School of Medicine

CHRISTINA STADLER, PhD
Professor for Developmental Psychiatry (Extraordinaria)
Department of Child and Adolescent Psychiatry
Psychiatric Clinics of the University of Basel

MICHAEL KELLY, MD
Clinical Assistant Professor
Division of Child and Adolescent Psychiatry
Stanford University School of Medicine

OXFORD
UNIVERSITY PRESS

OXFORD
UNIVERSITY PRESS

Oxford University Press is a department of the University of Oxford. It furthers
the University's objective of excellence in research, scholarship, and education
by publishing worldwide. Oxford is a registered trade mark of Oxford University
Press in the UK and certain other countries.

Published in the United States of America by Oxford University Press
198 Madison Avenue, New York, NY 10016, United States of America.

© Oxford University Press 2017

CIP data is on file at the Library of Congress
ISBN 978-0-19-026545-8

9 8 7 6 5 4 3 2 1

Printed by WebCom, Inc., Canada

Contents

Acknowledgments

I, Hans Steiner, would like to thank, first and foremost, my team of co-authors, who worked hard and diligently on bringing this book to completion. It has been heartening to see their energy and interest in this complex area of medicine. It is most gratifying to hand off to them all that I have learned in my 40 years of teaching, researching, and consulting to institutions and patients and their parents. They are a wonderful example of the type of individuals who will carry forth this important effort: to bring modern medicine with all its resources— diagnostic, therapeutic, and research—to a population that most people do not immediately see as deserving our dedication, because they have transgressed. It remains important to remember that even those who violate our rules of conviviality and civility may need the type of understanding and support modern medicine can offer. Being held accountable and confined is not enough.

I also would like to thank all my previous students who have helped me bring a substantial body of knowledge to this domain of research and teaching: Elizabeth Cauffman, PhD; Marina Zelenko, MD; Jeff Wilson, MD; Maya Petersen, MPH; Amy Campanaro, PhD; Belinda Plattner, MD; Sabine Voelkl-Kernstock, PhD; Melissa Silvermann, MD; Allison Redlich, PhD; Stephanie Hawkins, PhD; Laura Delizonna, PhD; Kirti Saxena, MD; Leena Khanzode, MD; Ranjit Padhy, MD; Marie Soller, MD; Arne Popma, MD; Niranjan Karnik, MD, PhD; Martin Fuchs, MD; Julia Huemer, MD.

My final thanks is to all the donors (S & T Geballe, P.K. Friedman) and funding agencies (National Institute of Justice, California Wellness Foundation, San Francisco Foundation, California Youth Authority) who have made most of this work possible. Without their unflagging support it would have been impossible to be part of the national group of scholars and researchers who have moved the field in very significant ways in the past 40 years.

I, Whitney Daniels, am so incredibly blessed with the opportunity to be surrounded by such a reinforcing team of co-authors that have demonstrated limitless patience, guidance, and enlightenment. For them, I am eternally grateful. While I hope I have made my family proud, I am immensely thankful to them, near and far, having supported me throughout this endeavor and during my career. I am indebted to the great and thoughtful teachers who have planted and nurtured the seeds of my education. Among them, Dr. Hans Steiner, Dr. Donald Knowlan, Dr. William Greenberg, Dr. Shashank Joshi, Dr. Carl Feinstein, Dr. Laura Roberts, Dr. Antonio Hardan, Dr. Manpreet Singh, Dr. Richard Shaw, Dr. Linda Lotspeich, Dr. Manasi Rana, Dr. Alan Louie, and Dr. Takesha Cooper. These are teachers who have seen me worthy of imparting their wisdom and knowledge, of which I am truly grateful. The patients and families who entrust their care to me deserve a great deal of acknowledgement, for they are my living, breathing textbooks. It is my hope that this literary contribution, returns even a fraction of what they have provided for the field.

I, Michael Kelly, would like to thank my co-authors, family, friends, and colleagues for their great support. I am especially grateful to Dr. Hans Steiner and the other teachers who have supported me along this path, including Jesse Velez, Pete Harames, Flo Kimmerling, Dr. Ze'ev Levin, Dr. Eve Caligor, Dr. Elizabeth Ford, Dr. Shashank Joshi, Dr. Antonio Hardan, Dr. Charles Scott, Dr. Barbara McDermott, Dr. Peter Ash, Dr. Alan Louie, and Dr. Laura Roberts. A special thank you to Drs. Anne McBride and John Hearn for their expert advice related to chapter 6 of this text. Also, a personal thank you to M.B. and P.H. Last, I would like to thank the patients and families with whom I work and learn from every day for allowing me to be a part of their lives.

I, Christina Stadler, first would like to thank Hans to give me the chance to take part in this great book project. Hans also is on the advisory board of our ongoing EU project FemNAT-CD "Neurobiology and Treatment of Adolescent Female Conduct Disorder: The Central Role of Emotion Processing," which is coordinated by Professor Christine Freitag whom I also would like to thank along with all the other researchers in this project, namely Prof. Arne Popma, Dr. Nauta-Jansen, Prof. Dr. Herpertz-Dahlmann, Prof. Kerstin Konrad, Dr. Graeme Fairchild, Dr. Stephane De Brito, Prof. Inga Neumann, Prof. Sabine Herpertz, Dr. Katja Bertsch, Prof. Meinhard Kieser, Prof. Araanzazu Fernandez Rivas, Dr. Agnes Vetro, Dr. Amaia Hervas, and Prof. Dimitris G. Dikeos.

I am especially grateful to my teacher, Fritz Poustka, who had strongly supported me on my scientific career in Frankfurt and to Prof. Robert Trestman Chair of Psychiatry at the Virginia Tech/Carilion School of Medicine and Carilion Clinic with whom our department has a fruitful cooperation within treatment research for disruptive behavior disorders.

Finally a special thanks to my team in Basel, Dr. Nora Raschle, Dr. Noortje Vriends, Dr. Martin Steppan, Dr. Margarete Bolten, Rebecca Mäkeläinen,

Dr. Ullrich Hildebrandt, Dr. Natalia Adamsi, and Dr. Barbara Rost and my PhD students Linda Kersten, Willeke Menks, Lynn Fehlbaum, Martin Prätzlich, and Dr. Felix Euler and all other students who contributed with their tremendous motivation and enthusiasm to bring us a step closer to our goal of understanding disruptive behavior disorders' etiology and developing treatment opportunities for our patients and their families.

1

Introduction to Disruptive Behavior Disorders

1.1 What Is the Problem?

Disruptive behavior disorders (DBDs) are among the most common diagnoses in mental health clinics. They constitute about 40% to 60% of referrals in clinics and practices helping children and adolescents with psychiatric problems. They are also commonly referred to under their subset labels: oppositional defiant disorder (ODD), conduct disorder (CD), and other specified and unspecified disruptive and impulse-control disorders. There have been some recent changes in the taxonomy of the American *Diagnostic and Statistical Manual of Mental Disorders* (5th ed.; DSM-5) and the International Classification of Diseases, which have implications for diagnosis and treatment that we discuss extensively.

DBDs are complex conditions that frequently co-occur with other diagnoses and/or are misdiagnosed all together. Youth with DBDs and their families often present to clinicians with maximal levels of dysfunction at home, school, work, and/or social environments. Very often, there is involvement with the law, especially in the adolescent age range. We believe that a developmental approach grounded in an understanding of behaviors suggestive of typical development and cognizant of symptoms indicating abnormal or atypical development is essential in accurately diagnosing and treating DBDs (Steiner, 2015). A developmental perspective is mindful of the context in which DBD symptoms arise (e.g., family structure, peer group, neighborhood, educational system) and their potential impact on the behavior of children. The developmental perspective presented in this text began its evolution during the nineteenth century, has matured over the years, and now rests on solid empirical data and practice-based evidence.

The birth of the child-saving movement during the nineteenth century, which occurred as a result of troubling events of the time and rapid increases in juvenile delinquency, was an early sign of a growing developmental perspective revolving around altruism and humanism. The Child Savers, especially Jane Addams, made their mark in the nineteenth century by petitioning for the development of a juvenile justice system—a system based primarily on young offenders' developmental status, not simply the types of crimes they committed and usual consequences. The Child Savers believed that focusing on youths' developmental status was essential for early identification and prevention. Such efforts consisted of educating and providing appropriate guidance to parents, other caregivers, and custodial and criminological personnel on normal and abnormal child development (Platt, 1977).

This Child Saving reform helped to establish the first juvenile court, located in Cook County, Illinois, in 1899, as a means of providing age-appropriate accountability, remediation, and rehabilitation. The process of establishing the first juvenile court was not without its growing pains. Among these challenges were unfair sentencing and arrests, which rose significantly despite the efforts of the reform. Additional backlash presented by way of overabundance of adult supervision. In another example, Addams spearheaded the creation of the Hull House, a settlement house located in Chicago, and later the Juvenile Protective Association whose mission was to curb juvenile delinquency throughout Chicago. Overall, the Child Savers movement generated a great deal of overdue attention to the topic of juvenile delinquency and led to new interventions for disenfranchised and at-risk youth.

A similar movement to that of the Chicago-based Child Savers emerged a few years later in Europe, under the direction of the director of the Vienna Juvenile Reform Schools in the 1920s and 1930s, August Aichhorn. Aichhorn sought to address the same concerns as the Child Savers with an educational/developmental approach. His theories and conceptualizations added a potentially valid treatment perspective to the forensic innovations of the Chicago reformers. Aichhorn was well acquainted with Sigmund Freud's writings and in close contact with the psychoanalytic community. He was first and foremost a teacher, who, with Anna Freud's encouragement, later became a psychoanalyst himself. Aichhorn (1935/1984) also published the seminal text *Verwahrloste Jugend* [*Wayward Youth*]. He was the first to approach juvenile delinquency from a developmental, psychiatric, psychological, and pedagogical perspective. Aichhorn's perspective strongly acknowledged the social context in which juvenile delinquency arose. According to Aichhorn, aggressive and antisocial behavior in youth was indicative of developmental trajectories gone awry. In Aichhorn's view, children start out in life as "asocial" beings whose world view does not extend beyond their own desires. As children grow, society demands that they develop a capacity to see beyond themselves, cope with frustration, and fulfill their needs while navigating the demands of others. According to Aichhorn, "The child needs to be educated into a state of prosocial adjustment, a task which only can be fulfilled if the child's emotional development proceeds normally." A major turning point in how we view the young people described in this text is credited to Aichhorn, who was the first to separate criminal labels from clinical ones. This change in perspective paved the way for studies of delinquents, aggression, and antisocial acts as forms of psychiatric syndromes, independent of court proceedings and adjudication. Aichhorn essentially founded the discipline of psychoeducation and child guidance. His philosophies have collectively influenced our field, ultimately laying the groundwork for the development of effective interventions informed by psychological and developmental principles.

Aichhorn's masterful depictions of youth in the early twentieth century mirror the harsh realities and associated emotional problems faced by many young people in modern society. His work has helped us understand much of what children in impoverished neighborhoods in the United States today are still experiencing. If we assume that the United States is historically rooted in violence, gun ownership, gang organizations, and a lack of social supports and structures, we can see how raising children under such circumstances is a formidable task. In his famous third chapter of *Wayward Youth*, Aichhorn presents an impressive array of case studies that link antisocial behaviors such as stealing, lying, aggression, and even violence to growing up in poverty. The children Aichhorn depicted lived in communities with inadequate schools, impoverished infrastructures, and regular exposure to potentially traumatic events, such as industrial and other accidents. Today, Aichhorn's Vienna of the 1920s is alive and well in places like East Los Angeles, New Orleans, Oakland, San Jose, and Washington, DC, to name a few. While the approaches to addressing aggression and antisocial behavior in youth have evolved over time, we value and share the developmental perspective pioneered by the Child Savers and August Aichhorn nearly a century ago. Aichhorn's work spawned a growing stream of clinical, epidemiological, basic scientific, and, most recently, neuroscientific studies that are the backbone of this volume.

1.2 Why Have We Been So Slow in Moving the Field?

An explanatory note is called for at this point. As mentioned, the majority of youth treated in child and adolescent psychiatry clinics throughout North America will have problems related to some form of aggression. We still struggle, however, with diagnosis and specific treatment for these youths. We have had the developmental and pedagogic perspective on these problems for many years without the rapid progress in identification, prevention, and treatment we should hope for. The study of aggression and mental disorders, in which aggression is a hallmark feature (e.g., CD, ODD), lags behind that of other areas of child and adolescent psychiatry (e.g., attention deficit hyperactivity disorder [ADHD], anxiety, depression). To what can this delay and slowed progress be attributed? In our view, the reasons for the relatively slow progress in the study of aggression and its associated conditions are complex historical, political, and methodological. Antisocial acts and aggression, which constitute the main cluster of symptoms in this grouping of disorders, are very common, especially in the adolescent age range and in toddlerhood. This can be confusing in attempting to delineate normal from pathological development. Also contributing to the difficulty with diagnosing these disorders is the fact, that by definition, most of these acts involve other people—one person's aggression is another's standing up for oneself in self-defense—and societal norms. The latter certainly vary widely, especially with large countries, like the United States; countries that are diverse in their population characteristics; or countries that are in chaos, such as during wartime. All of these factors contribute to problems with accurate identification and measurement of response to intervention. Unlike almost exclusively based internalizing syndromes, such as depression, we have to struggle as clinicians to do the best we can do under very complicated circumstances.

Another reason that is more of a political nature probably also contributed to the current state of affairs. In 1988, Vice President George H. W. Bush appointed Dr. Fredrick Goodwin to head the Alcohol, Drug Abuse, and Mental Health Administration (ADAMHA). Goodwin was a proponent of the Violence Initiative, a federal proposal by the department of Health and Human Services that sought to reduce violent crime in America's inner cities by identifying individuals, primarily inner-city youths, whose background and genetic makeup placed them at risk for committing unlawful acts of aggression. The hope of those involved in creating the Violence Initiative was that identifying at-risk youth would lead to effective early intervention and ultimately reduce inner-city violence. During a 1992 press conference, Goodwin likened the "loss of social structure" within "high impact inner-city areas" prone to violence to the behavior of monkeys in the wild. Goodwin's comments sparked a firestorm of controversy and fears by some that the government would use the Violence Initiative as a means of controlling disenfranchised youth deemed at risk for violence through psychotropic medications. Goodwin resigned from his position as head of the ADAMHA shortly after making these remarks, the Violence Initiative faded from public view, and federally funded studies of aggression became politically risky. This discouraged young researchers from pursuing the topic, national agencies such as the National Institute of Mental Health (NIMH) from funding studies, and industry from investment in developing and researching medications that could contribute to successful treatment. The end result was a hiatus of several decades, during which this important area of clinical child and adolescent psychiatry languished.

In recent years, the study of antisocial acts, aggression, and its antecedents has been resurrected in the United States due to exciting emerging evidence from neuroscience, epidemiology, and clinical trials. For instance, the pioneering work of James Blair at the NIMH has elucidated the neurobiological underpinnings of psychopathy and aggression leading to initiatives like the NIMH proposed Research Domain Criteria (RDoC) approach (Blair, Karnik, Coccaro, & Steiner, 2009). The RDoC provides a dimensional perspective, steering the field away from the current categorical perspective espoused by the DSM. In addition, research over the past 20 years has identified distinct subtypes of aggression (e.g., predatory vs. reactive) based on neurocognitive underpinnings of disruptive behavior that have major implications on the effectiveness of psychotherapeutic and medication interventions (Blair et al., 2009; Padhy et al., 2011; Steiner, 1999; Steiner & Karnik, 2004; Vitiello, Behar, Hunt, Stoff, & Ricciuti, 1990; Vitiello & Stoff, 1997).

The work of Hans Eysenk, Adrian Raine, James Blair, Paul Frick, Robert Hare, and members of their laboratories and clinics over the past 20 years has significantly advanced our understanding of aggression and antisocial behavior. However, our current diagnostic scheme, the DSM-5, has not thoroughly integrated the remarkable insights of August Aichhorn's developmental perspective, innovative approaches such as the RDoC dimensional based approach, or accumulating data on the neurobiology of aggression with its conceptualization of youth aggression and antisocial behavior. The DSM-5 lists a variety of symptoms for disorders associated with pathological aggression, most notably CD and ODD. By contrast, a truly developmental psychiatry perspective on dissocial behavior and the latest research findings suggests that whether these behaviors are truly "symptoms" of an internally based disorder are best understood when the context (e.g., social environment, past experiences, temperament) in which they occur has been taken into account and ruled out as the major driver of the problem. From a developmental psychiatry perspective, DBDs are not always intrinsically determined, as the criteria set forth by the DSM-5 implies. For instance, socioeconomic and ethnic bias is a flaw within our current classification system for DBDs.

This is relevant, because, for instance, our juvenile justice system has disproportionate numbers of youth who come from poor backgrounds and ethnic minorities. Most of the youth involved in the American juvenile justice system, a population of high ecological validity, meet criteria for some form of DBD. The lopsided nature of the population within our juvenile justice system is testament to the fact that, in general, DBD diagnoses are not fixed innate genetically predetermined conditions. Instead, the development of DBDs is influenced by a wide variety of psychosocial risk factors (e.g., peer group, family system, socio-economic status, temperament, genetic background).

As illustrative examples, let us consider a scenario where a youth lives in an active warzone or is a refugee fighting for survival. Acts of stealing, deception, lying, robbery, and even aggression assume a very different meaning when we find ourselves in such circumstances. To diagnose a youth with CD while he is fighting for survival would indeed be adding insult to injury. We contend that by focusing on the environmental, biological, and underlying neurocognitive factors that influence aggression we can better delineate the syndromes that truly are predominantly internally driven. That is, we can begin to describe the aspects of youth's presentation that operate somewhat independently of social context (e.g., temperament, biologic reactivity) and implement individualized treatment approaches that are consistent with current theories on child development and the latest research (Padhy et al., 2011).

Starting with the third edition of the DSM in 1980, classifying aggression and antisocial acts according to diagnostic criteria was a significant step forward in helping clinicians identify patients and their needs, independent of the juvenile justice system. We discuss the exact criteria for classification of DBDs in the DSM and the International Classification of Diseases in chapter 2. In the meantime, we offer another important critique of the current diagnostic practices. Additionally, we propose an alternate clinical template that is based on the integration of findings from clinical and preclinical studies and takes into account the problems that arise when we ignore social context. Our current classification system includes few important distinctions of the type of aggression and antisocial acts that have shown promise in developing a more refined diagnostic approach and allow for more precisely tailored interventions.

Before we discuss the state of diagnosis (chapter 2), epidemiology (chapter 3), etiology (chapter 4), and treatment (chapter 5), as well as the implications of our knowledge for forensic populations (chapter 6), we offer a carefully considered list of criticisms of the way we diagnose DBDs at the present time. This will help us stay abreast of the field and will instill us with appropriate caution as we approach this difficult set of problems.

1.3 Persistent Problems with Current Psychiatric Approaches to Antisocial and Aggressive Acts and Possible Solutions

The current diagnostic criteria in the DSM-5 do not differentiate youth based on their profile of aggression. We have come to appreciate that aggression and antisocial behavior can either be carefully planned or can be highly reactive to triggers and circumstances. In the 1980s, a workgroup assembled by the American Academy of Child & Adolescent Psychiatry at Howard University, under the leadership of Stanford University, used the opinions of well-known experts in the fields of research, clinical practice, and teaching to propose a schema that rested on a broad collection of preclinical, clinical, and neuroscientific studies. The workgroup differentiated planned (Proactive/Instrumental/Predatory) and emotionally reactive (Reactive/Affective/Defensive/Impulsive) acts of aggression (Steiner, 2011). Making such distinctions begins to acknowledge the heterogeneity within youth who meet criteria for diagnoses like CD and ODD. Different subtypes of aggression and their associate behaviors run on distinct neuroscientific mechanisms, which are part of either the highest level of cerebral functioning (as in the case of proactive/instrumental/planned [PIP]) or part of the threat/alarm system (as in the case of reactive/affective/defensive/impulsive [RADI]) and often require different forms of intervention (Connor, Glatt, Lopez, Jackson, & Melloni, 2002). Because these subtypes of symptoms are usually not separated and targeted specifically, it should come as no surprise that most of our clinical trials to date have shown only modest to moderate effects. We have demonstrated this by a reanalysis of one of our own clinical trials (Padhy et al., 2011), where disaggregation of these subtypes strengthened the outcome of the double-blind placebo-controlled medication considerably. The "symptoms" listed in the DSM-5 are sets of behaviors that can result from a variety of etiologies and be easily attributed to either of these subtypes. For instance, a youth can steal because he has been stolen from and feels justified in his rage about that fact. The resultant theft would be attributable to a RADI subtype of aggression. Another youth can carefully plan and implement the theft of a cell phone from a classmate who has never done anything to him. The goal of this act is acquisition, while carefully avoiding detection. This would represent a PIP subtype. The former would probably benefit from medications that keep emotions under control, but the latter most likely would not. Given the current limitations of our diagnostic approach, it is difficult to recommend specific treatment plans based on a DBD diagnosis alone. Adding other specifiers—such as age of onset, callous-unemotional dimensions, and the PIP/RADI label—is usually necessary and potentially beneficial.

A serious criticism of DBD diagnoses in their current configuration is the lack of positive predictive validity. The stability of DBD diagnoses over time in youth ranging from preschool to late adolescents and adulthood tend to vary greatly depending on the type of instrument used, the population studied, and the version of diagnostic criteria used. For example, based on the current classification system within the DSM-5, we are not able to predict with much accuracy from any particular symptom in the diagnostic criteria array which youth with DBDs will go on to develop antisocial personality disorder, starting in childhood moving forward to young adulthood. This implies that there is a subcohort of youth with DBDs that we are inadequately identifying by the use of the current criteria (Steiner & Remsing, 2007). Based on what we know now, it is not possible to predict who will ultimately exit from such a diagnosis or progress into increasingly severe subtypes (ODD to CD to antisocial personality disorder) going into young adulthood. While the current criteria offer solid evidence for separate clinicians, agreeing that such symptoms are present (concurrent validity), the implications of such an agreement for the future are not clear. This is of course a problem, as one tries to detect, intervene, and heal. For instance, to intervene may or may not be in fact necessary, or failure to intervene may confer increasing chronicity and problems.

An additional concern is that the current process of defining and redefining DBDs and their subtypes often results in a proliferation of diagnoses of questionable utility, before we even have made sure that the basic categories of diagnoses (CD, ODD) are firmly established. Everyone has witnessed the progressive growth of the DSM over the decades, which has been criticized by many and has resulted in the nickname of "the book of names" in some critics' writings. As an example, the current version of the DSM contains a new diagnosis called disruptive mood dysregulation disorder (DMDD). DMDD was created as a means of preventing the overdiagnosis of pediatric bipolar disorder. While in some ways, this is a small step in the right direction, through integration of RADI and PIP divisions into diagnoses, we still encounter major problems. The symptoms for DMDD are nonspecific, and the disorder itself is highly correlated with DBDs; yet the diagnosis of DMDD is less stable over time than DBDs (Axelson, 2013; Axelson et al., 2012). Moreover, the diagnosis is in its infancy, and there are no clear treatment guidelines (Roy, Lopes, & Klein, 2014). We contend that because there are a number of pathways to reaching the criteria for DMDD, the diagnosis can mislead or complicate the direction of treatment for the young people we serve, unless we refine it and bring to bear our insights from the RADI/PIP distinction.

These critiques have implications affecting medical treatment options. In regard to medications, there are currently no drug indications for DBDs. This may be due in part to the lack of financial incentive to perform clinical trials involving drugs thought to curb aggression, most if not all of which have generic alternatives. However, there is some very good evidence from a meta-analysis that stimulant medications can curb overt "hot" aggression in youth with ADHD (Connor et al., 2002) more so than covert "cold" aggression. As we mentioned previously, a reanalysis of our randomized controlled trial by Padhy and colleagues (2011) looked at youth with both hot and cold CD in youth and found that roughly half of youth prone to hot aggression had reductions in aggressive behavior in response to valproic acid (Depakote). The majority of youth prone to cold aggression showed no response in their levels of aggression in response to medications. Furthermore, among the youth prone to hot aggression, their reductions in aggressive behavior reduced by twice as much in response to higher doses of medications, unlike those who engaged in cold aggression, who were relatively impervious to the effects of medications to curb aggression.

Another excellent example of factors that might lead us in a more fruitful direction in our diagnostic attempts are the recent data describing biological characteristics that put people at risk for maladaptive forms of cold aggression and psychopathy. According to the work of Hans Eysenk and his protégée Adrian Raine, low autonomic arousal in response to stress is a risk factor for cold aggression (Raine, 2015) These findings have not been received without controversy and vigorous debate, but they are based on a series of longitudinal follow-up from infancy to adolescence and beyond, complemented by findings from experimental studies that are extremely persuasive in their coherence and consistency.

Another set of studies has been stimulated by the progressive growth of cognitive neuroscience, a branch of the neurosciences that seeks to link behavioral observations to basic brain processes to inform our understanding of psychopathology. For instance, Blair (2004, 2016) has been able to identify other important neurocognitive factors that shed light on the psychological dysfunctions in psychopathic individuals and actually open the door for future novel intervention programs. For one, such individuals have a lack of empathic response to other people's injury, anxiety, and pain; for another, they are deficient in altering their response to adverse outcomes as the odds increase that they will not achieve desired goals. They will persist in taking unusual risks, even when the odds have been experimentally changed so that a negative outcome is virtually guaranteed (Blair, 2004; Blair, 2016). It stands to reason that when such individuals are raised in a warm, loving, and supportive environment, they can go on to overcome such tendencies and become productive members of society. However, when youth with these traits are raised in a violent environment with harsh discipline and inconsistent or absent parenting, we set the stage for youth who see violence as a productive tool, an instrument for acquisition and dominance. These then become individuals who ultimately account for a substantial portion of the criminal misery in our society.

1.4 The Structure of This Book

In this volume we offer a carefully considered selective review of the most recent literature on the subject of DBDs. We make every possible attempt to capture the essence of the scientific literature without derailing into a pedantic academic-type discussion of controversies and deficiencies. The general tone of this volume is aimed at the front-line clinician and young researcher. But while we are smoothing the peaks and valleys of disagreements, we hope to preserve the critical posture that is appropriate when a field is engaged in rapid growth and resulting unevenness.

Each chapter offers a definition of the subject area discussed, a review of the most current literature, a summary of controversies and open questions, necessary next steps to move the field, the implications for private practice, and a list of references cited, followed by suggested further readings, Web, and community resources. The chapters discuss taxonomy, classification and diagnosis, etiology, epidemiology, comprehensive integrated treatment, and the implications of our current knowledge for the theory and practice of forensic psychiatry and criminology.

It is our hope that this book will provide insights into the nature of aggression and its manifestations, furthering the discussion of how we can best address the needs of at-risk youth around the world. There is much movement in preclinical, basic, epidemiological, clinical, and preventive research that should make us hopeful that the next generation of clinicians, patients, and parents will face considerably better odds to achieve good outcomes. We hope to provide readers with the basis for such optimism and to attract the best and the brightest to work on these complex problems.

References

Aichhorn, A. (1984). *Wayward Youth*. Evanston, IL: Northwestern University Press. (Original work published 1935), 14.

Axelson, D. (2013). Taking disruptive mood dysregulation disorder out for a test drive. *American Journal of Psychiatry*, 170(2), 136–139.

Axelson, D., Findling, R. L., Fristad, M. A., Kowatch, R. A., Youngstrom, E. A., Horwitz, S. M., . . . Demeter, C. (2012). Examining the proposed disruptive mood dysregulation disorder diagnosis in children in the Longitudinal Assessment of Manic Symptoms study. *Journal of Clinical Psychiatry*, 73(10), 1342–1350.

Blair, R. (2004). The roles of orbital frontal cortex in the modulation of antisocial behavior. *Brain and Cognition*, 55(1), 198–208.

Blair, R. J. (2016). The neurobiology of impulsive aggression. *Journal of Child and Adolescent Psychopharmacology*, 26(1), 4–9.

Blair, J., Karnik, N. S., Coccaro, E., & Steiner, H. (2009). Taxonomy and neurobiology of aggression. In E. P. Benedek, P. Ash, & C. L. Scott (Eds.), *Principles and practice of child and adolescent forensic mental health* (pp. 267–278). Washington, DC: American Psychiatric Publishing.

Connor, D. F., Glatt, S. J., Lopez, I. D., Jackson, D., & Melloni, R. H. (2002). Psychopharmacology and aggression. I: A meta-analysis of stimulant effects on overt/covert aggression–related behaviors in ADHD. *Journal of the American Academy of Child & Adolescent Psychiatry, 41*(3), 253–261.

Padhy, R., Saxena, K., Remsing, L., Huemer, J., Plattner, B., & Steiner, H. (2011). Symptomatic response to divalproex in subtypes of conduct disorder. *Child Psychiatry & Human Development, 42*(5), 584–593.

Raine, A. (2015). Low resting heart rate as an unequivocal risk factor for both the perpetration of and exposure to violence. *JAMA Psychiatry, 72*(10), 962–964. doi:10.1001/jamapsychiatry.2015.1364

Roy, A. K., Lopes, V., & Klein, R. G. (2014). Disruptive mood dysregulation disorder: A new diagnostic approach to chronic irritability in youth. *The American Journal of Psychiatry, 171*(9), 918–924.

Steiner, H. (1999). Disruptive behavior disorders. In H. I. Kaplan & B. J. Sadock (Eds.), *Comprehensive textbook of psychiatry* (Vol. VII, pp. 2693–2704). New York: Lippincott Williams & Wilkins.

Steiner, H., Cauffman, E., & Duxbury, E. (1999). Personality traits in juvenile delinquents: Relation to criminal behavior and recidivism. *Journal of the American Academy of Child & Adolescent Psychiatry, 38*(3), 256–262. doi:10.1097/00004583-199903000-00011

Steiner, H., & Karnik, N. (2004). Child or adolescent antisocial behavior. In B. J. Sadock & V. A. Sadock (Eds.), *Comprehensive textbook of psychiatry/VIII* (Vol. 2, pp. 1415–1432). New York: Williams & Wilkins.

Steiner, H., & Remsing, L. (2007). Practice parameter for the assessment and treatment of children and adolescents with oppositional defiant disorder. *Journal of the American Academy of Child & Adolescent Psychiatry, 46*(1), 126–141.

Vitiello, B., Behar, D., Hunt, J., Stoff, D., & Ricciuti, A. (1990). Subtyping aggression in children and adolescents. *Journal of Neuropsychiatry and Clinical Neurosciences, 2*(2), 189–192.

Vitiello, B., & Stoff, D. M. (1997). Subtypes of aggression and their relevance to child psychiatry. *Journal of the American Academy of Child & Adolescent Psychiatry, 36*(3), 307–315.

Suggested Reading and Resources

Platt, A. (1977). *Child Savers* (2nd ed.). Chicago: University of Chicago Press.

Raine, A. (2013). *The anatomy of violence: The biological roots of crime.* New York: Vintage.

Steiner, H. (2011). *Handbook of developmental psychiatry.* Singapore: World Scientific.

Steiner, H. (2015). *Treating adolescents.* Hoboken, NJ: John Wiley.

Books for Parents

Fabiano, G. A. (2016). *Interventions for disruptive behaviors: Reducing problems and building skills.* New York: Guilford Press.

Greene, R. W. (2009). *Lost at school: Why our kids with behavioral challenges are falling through the cracks and how we can help them.* New York: Simon & Schuster.

Gresham, F. M. (2015). *Disruptive behavior disorders: Evidence-based practice for assessment and intervention.* New York: Guilford Press.

Walls, S. (2016). *Oppositional defiant & disruptive children and adolescents: Non-medication approaches for the most challenging ODD behaviors.* Eau Claire, WI: PESI.

2

Taxonomy, Classification, and Diagnosis of Disruptive Behavior Disorders

In order to be as well prepared as possible for the complex topic of disruptive behavior disorders (DBDs), we start by dedicating some thought and discussion to DBDs and their taxonomy. A thoughtful approach to diagnosis is crucial in medicine, because establishing diagnoses are the initial steps in determining a patient's comprehensive evaluation and treatment plan. Well-thought-out diagnostic formulations are an especially important issue for youth with DBDs due to these disorders' clinical complexity and existing shortcomings of the current diagnostic nomenclature. DBD symptoms are interpersonal and multilayered, making them difficult to exactly pinpoint and categorize. Additionally, the DBD diagnostic grouping is a relatively new addition to our diagnostic classification schemes. DBDs have been described in clinical textbooks and the target of research for about 80 years. That said, they have been the subject of intense study for only around 40 years, since the advent of the third edition of the *Diagnostic and Statistical Manual of Mental Disorders* (DSM). DBDs are relative newcomers whose literature base pales in comparison to the study of psychotic anxiety and depressive disorders, which have been studied for centuries in one form or another.

As discussed in chapter 1, the idea that problems with impulsivity, aggression, violence, and antisocial behavior could benefit from a noncriminological, medical, developmental, and psychological perspective is relatively new. Such ideas regarding DBDs are have not always appealed to lay people or lawyers, judges, and justice personnel. As we will see in chapter 6, the introduction of these disorders raises important questions within the domain of our criminal and juvenile justice systems (e.g., how much do these diagnoses exculpate the patient from being held accountable for his or her actions? How much is an individual in charge of his or her actions and how much are these driven by some disorder or dysfunction?). The multiplicity of current terms applied to these problems in psychiatry poses a challenge to the student, practitioner, and researcher. We enumerate these challenges and shed light on their relative importance and their impact on clinical practice.

2.1 Definitions

As discussed in chapter 1, we begin every chapter in this textbook with a list of definitions of terms used. We continue to follow this practice throughout the book in order to eradicate idiosyncrasies in readers' thinking. Such a recapitulation of terms is especially necessary in the domain of DBDs because there are many lay and criminological terms that overlap with psychopathological definitions, sometimes causing confusion in the minds of even the most studious and learned among us. Furthermore, as also will become clear as we progress, there are often differences in the ways that researchers and clinicians define terms relevant to DBDs. Sometimes these discrepancies are not just confusion but reflect progress in the field that has not completely trickled down to the practitioner or bubbled up from clinical practice to the scientists.

Diagnosis: "the determination of the nature of a disease; a deciding" (Stedman 2006).

Diagnoses are categorical, syndromal types. These types are a convenient way of summarizing a multiplicity of details about patients to facilitate communication with patients, their families, other doctors and professionals, and insurance companies. Ideally, they also relate to basic and advanced research in the field, guiding clinicians in a definitive direction as they plan treatment. Diagnoses are often presumed to be the main reason for the patient's need for health care services. As we will see in chapters 4 and 5, the current DBD diagnoses are limited in their power to suggest and lead us to specific and appropriate treatments. There is another possible distinction: for pragmatic purposes, diagnoses can also be divided into principal (or primary) diagnoses and secondary ones. Stedman (2006) gives us the following definitions:

Primary and secondary diagnosis: "the first or foremost of a disease or a group of symptoms to which others may be secondary or occur as complications."

We have previously published an account of how the concept of primary and secondary diagnoses may map onto DBDs (Steiner, Saxena, & Chang, 2004). The purpose of having clinicians determine a *primary diagnosis* is to establish where the bulk of clinical resources should be applied to heal a disease at a given point in its course. A primary diagnosis can occur in conjunction with underlying conditions that are difficult to treat. An example in the case of DBDs would be a patient with the primary diagnosis of conduct disorder (CD), complicated by substance use disorders and withdrawal symptoms. Despite CD predating the drug abuse, withdrawal symptoms can be severe enough that the focus of care (the primary diagnosis) shifts most resources to the management of the substance withdrawal rather than the antisocial behavior leading up to drug abuse (e.g., the sale of drugs to support one's own use or prostitution to maintain a regular supply of drugs). The chronic nature of these conditions shifts to the background (they become a secondary disorder), which will be targeted once the patient's primary disorder (withdrawal from opioids) is under control. Another label often applied is *principal diagnosis,* which is equivalent to primary diagnosis. As we will see, when we discuss the current cluster of DBDs in the fifth edition of the DSM (DSM-5), the new grouping contains several disorders that could all qualify for being a primary diagnosis, in principle. Whether or not they in fact are fulfilling this task adequately remains an open question. Ideally, diagnostic criteria should be specific enough to lead to a conclusive diagnosis. At this point it is not clear that any diagnoses in the DBD cluster are up to that standard.

Polithetic taxon: a cluster of critical and auxiliary symptoms, not just on a single symptom alone. Ideally, diagnoses should be based on more than one criterion (see the discussion of the Rosenhan experiment).

Both the DSM and the International Classification of Diseases (ICD) rely on lists of presumptive specific symptoms and symptom clusters as reported by the patient, people in their lives (e.g., friends, family), and/or treatment providers. The lists are then assigned thresholds leading to an algorithm that is assumed to lead to a diagnosis. At present, the rationale behind the cut-offs used to determine whether someone meets criteria for a DBD are uncertain. Thus our current diagnostic schemes cause clinicians who diagnose DBDs to face considerable uncertainty in regard to their etiology, needed treatment plan, and prognosis.

Supposedly, in the field trials of the DSM, for instance, there was systematic testing of the cohesion of specific diagnostic criteria in order to form a diagnostic cluster; however, nothing has been made public regarding these statistics. In fact, a great deal of criticism has been leveled at the science backing DSM diagnoses, for instance as manifested in the weak cohesion statistics for many diagnoses. At the present time it is not possible to know whether the DBDs are affected by this problem, as there are no data available. Our best guess is that there should be adequate concurrent validity but unknown external (i.e., they apply to patients in the real world) and prospective (i.e., they predict what will happen in the natural course of a particular disorder) validity, as has been the case with previous iterations of the DBD diagnoses. This means that while applying the criteria of DBDs as specified by the DSM will generate some reasonable agreement between independent raters that a diagnosis is present, there is little or no support for any prediction of treatment need and response and future course of illness or recovery. This will become more evident in chapters 3 and 5, as we look at the natural progression of DBD disorders and treatment of them.

Disorder: "a disturbance of function, structure or both resulting from a failure in development or from exogenous factors such as poison, trauma or disease" (Stedman, 2006).

This is a more general label than a disease. It usually denotes a clinical state where we are uncertain as to the exact diagnosis and the underlying causal processes, but we acknowledge that the condition brings on dysfunction and suffering. The DSM and ICD systems label such states "other specified disruptive, impulse-control, and conduct disorder," where the clinician lists the diagnostic criteria missing to assign a more definitive diagnosis, and an "unspecified disruptive, impulse-control, and conduct disorder" (see Box 2.1), which gives the clinician more latitude in listing the missing criteria. These diagnoses can be applied due to time pressure or to protect the patient from injudiciously incriminating him- or herself while in a justice setting where the reported criterion would lead to criminal consequences (e.g., the criterion of "arguing with authority figures" in oppositional defiant disorder [ODD] or the criterion of "stealing items of non-trivial value without confronting a victim") Such a category also helps the clinician refrain from jumping to conclusions while trying to build rapport with a juvenile.

Box 2.1 **Disruptive, Impulse-Control, and Conduct Disorders**

Oppositional defiant disorder (313.81; ICD-10 F91.3)

Conduct disorder (312.81; ICD-10 F91.1—childhood onset, 312.32; ICD-10 F91.2 adolescent onset, and 312.89; ICD-10 F91.9—unspecified onset)

Otherwise specified disruptive, impulse-control, and conduct disorder category, where some criteria are missing, as listed by the clinician (312.89; ICD-10 F91.8)

Unspecified disruptive impulse-control and conduct disorder, where the clinician elects not to report the missing criteria (312.9; ICD-10 F91.9)

Intermittent explosive disorder (312.34; ICD-10 F63.81)

Pyromania (312.33; ICD-10 F63.1)

Kleptomania (312.32; ICD-10 F63.3)

Antisocial personality disorder (301.7; ICD-10 F60.2), also listed under Cluster B Personality Disorders)

It is not only in DBDs where such diagnostic caution is helpful. Another example would be in the category of substance use disorder, whose diagnostic criteria ipso facto are against the law by virtue of the patient's age. In our studies with juvenile justice populations, we decided to change the time frame of drug use reporting to events occurring only prior to incarceration and adjudication, assuring that the youths would receive some protection while still allowing us to draw some diagnostic conclusions. We resume this discussion in chapter 6 when we focus on the forensic implications of this diagnostic grouping.

Disease: "a morbid entity characterized usually by at least two of these criteria: recognized etiologic agent(s), identifiable group of signs and symptoms, or consistent anatomical alterations"(Stedman, 2006).

In contradistinction to disorder, this label requires greater certainty regarding the problem and goes beneath the surface, listing specific causal pathogenetic processes. Very few psychiatric disorders are in this "disease" category. DBDs in the present diagnostic configurations are not, as they lack the exact etiologic agent(s) and consistent anatomical alterations. They do possess identifiable symptoms (subjective patient reports) and some signs, as will become evident in our later discussion.

Differential diagnosis: "the determination of which of two or more diseases is the one from which the patient is suffering"(Stedman, 2006).

Differential diagnosis refers to the listing of the possible diagnoses that describe a given clinical presentation, which then are reduced to a primary diagnosis by a process of careful elimination. In essence, a differential diagnosis casts a wide net when considering how to classify an illness or set of behaviors. In a perfect scenario, as the criteria for defining a clinical presentation become more exact, we can begin eliminating candidates from our "differential," ultimately arriving at a single diagnosis. Such an endpoint is very desirable, as it should lead the clinician to a set of specific interventions with a high likelihood of positive outcomes. As we will see in chapter 5, discussing treatment, we are very often not so fortunate to arrive at one single diagnosis in the case of DBDs.

Comorbidity: "a concomitant but unrelated pathologic or disease process; usually used in epidemiology to indicate the coexistence of two or more disease processes" (Stedman, 2006).

Comorbidity refers to the presence of multiple disorders, thought to be separate and unrelated, impacting the same individual. For example, when we say that CD and substance use disorders are highly comorbid, we are saying that a large percentage of patients with CD also meet DSM-5 criteria for a substance use disorder. This immediately raises a question: As most activities during drug use in juveniles (using, acquiring, etc.) are ipso facto illegal, should they perhaps be part of the DBD diagnoses? Would it not be better, for instance, to create a subtype of CD with or without substance use and abuse of varying severity?

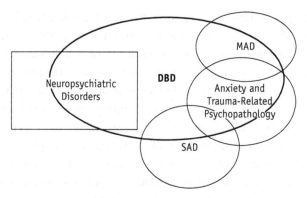

Figure 2.1 Comorbidity of the current DBD grouping: internalizing, externalizing, and neuropsychiatric disorders.

A severe case of substance use could be made a truly separate condition, as it requires more and different resources to treat it in addition to the conduct problems. Such overlaps with other conditions are extremely common in DBDs (see chapter 3 on epidemiology); in addition, as we will see in chapter 6, discussing forensics, the overlap between DBDs and other psychiatric problems in our studies of delinquents is extremely high, surpassing the counts usually found in clinical populations. Figure 2.1 is a schematic of what in various studies of DBDs has been found to be comorbid with them. We can see that this indeed is a very wide range of disorders, from neuropsychiatric disturbances to mood and anxiety diagnoses.

In part, this is most likely an artifact of the DSM system, which more so than the ICD system permits and even encourages the diagnosis of comorbidity. The danger of this approach is the tendency for clinicians to be content with simply tacking on several diagnoses, without much thought given to what might be the primary or secondary condition. In many practices, such an approach rapidly progresses to unfounded and even problematic polypharmacology, with all the difficulties this entails. This problem is not unique to DBDs. Examples across the DSM include considerable overlap between major depressive disorder and generalized anxiety disorder, or disruptive mood dysregulation disorder and ODD, to name a few.

As we started to ask, when such an overlap occurs with some regularity, can we really be sure that these comorbid disorders are not just part of the same overall syndrome rather than additional, discrete mental disorders? And what is the clinician to do at this point when faced with these overlaps and constant co-occurrences? We discuss some possible strategies in the clinical implications section at the end of this chapter. To hint at some of them, we discuss the ordering of the emergence points of different syndromes or disorders, as has been suggested by many developmental psychopathologists. There are also incipient changes within the DSM and the ICD systems that are somewhat helpful. The ICD in particular has introduced several possible subtypes that can be clinically useful in drawing these distinctions (see Tables 2.1 and 2.2), allowing subtypes based on socialized–unsocialized aspects of DBDs, anxiety, and mood; learning and its problems; and focus and its problems. It makes more sense of these variables used in the ICD simply as vehicles for subtyping DBDs, which only in rare cases would assume the status of truly separate diagnostic entities.

Table 2.1 **Comparing the Grouping of DBDs in the DSM-5 and ICD-10**

DSM-5 DBD Classification	ICD-10 DBD Classification
Disruptive, impulse-control, and conduct disorders	**Behavioral and emotional disorders with onset usually occurring in childhood and adolescence**
313.81 Oppositional Defiant Disorder	*F90 Hyperkinetic disorders*
312.34 Intermittent Explosive Disorder	F90.0 Disturbance of activity and attention
312.81 Conduct Disorder Childhood onset type	F90.1 Hyperkinetic conduct disorder
	F90.8 Other hyperkinetic disorders
312.82 Conduct Disorder Adolescent onset type	F90.9 Hyperkinetic disorder, unspecified
312.89 Conduct Disorder Unspecified onset (specify if with limited prosocial emotions; specify current severity: mild, moderate, severe)	*F91 Conduct disorders*
	F91.0 Conduct disorder confined to the family context
301.7 Antisocial Personality Disorder	F91.1 Unsocialized conduct disorder
312.33 Pyromania	F91.2 Socialized conduct disorder
312.32 Kleptomania	F91.3 Oppositional defiant disorder
312.89 Other Specified Disruptive, Impulse-Control, and Conduct Disorder	F91.8 Other conduct disorders
	F91.9 Conduct disorder, unspecified
	F92 Mixed disorders of conduct and emotions
	F92.0 Depressive conduct disorder
312.9 Unspecified Disruptive, Impulse-Control, and Conduct Disorder	F92.8 Other mixed disorders of conduct and emotions
	F92.9 Mixed disorder of conduct and emotions, unspecified

Note: DBD = disruptive behavior disorders; DSM-5 = *Diagnostic and Statistical Manual of Mental Disorders* (fifth edition); ICD-10 = International Classification of Diseases (tenth revision).

Table 2.2 Comparison of Specific Diagnostic Conduct Disorder Criteria and Subtypes DSM-5 and ICD-10: An Illustration of Differences

Conduct Disorder DSM-5 Criteria	Conduct Disorder ICD-10 Criteria
Childhood onset— before 10 years of age	➤ 3 of 15 criteria present in the past 12 months with at least one being present in the past 6 months
Adolescent onset—after age 10	• Arson participation
Severity Markers: mild, moderate, severe	• Destruction of property
	• Breaking curfew by age 13
DSM specific	• Running away from home for a significant period of time
Callous–unemotional specifier	• Persistent truancy before age 13
	• "Breaking and entering"
	• Lying for secondary gain
	• Stealing
	• Employed a serious weapon
	• Forced sexual acts on another
	• Stealing through face to face intimidation
	• Animal cruelty
	• Human cruelty
	• Frequent fight initiation
	• Frequent bullying
	Childhood onset—before 10 years of age
	Adolescent onset—after age 10
	Severity Markers: mild, moderate, severe
	ICD specific:
	Conduct disorder confined to family context—"Familial"—symptoms present when interacting with family
	Unsocialised conduct disorder—child does not have peer relationships or friends
	Socialised conduct disorder—child does have friends and peer relationships
	Depressive conduct disorder
	Hyperkinetic conduct disorder

Note: DSM-5 = *Diagnostic and Statistical Manual of Mental Disorders* (fifth edition); ICD-10 = International Classification of Diseases (tenth revision)

The DSM has fewer subtypes, using age and the callous–emotional dimensions as examples. Age has an immediate impact on the management of DBDs: the type of treatment chosen (home visitation, parent effectiveness training, anger management, or multisystemic family therapy would be good examples as we go from preschool to school age to adolescence; see the more detailed discussion in chapter 5 on treatment); callous–unemotional traits similarly have direct impact on treatment (see chapter 5 on treatment and chapter 4 on etiology).

Age-related presentations of disorders present another theoretical shift within our field with important implications: Increasingly, discussions have centered on clustering disorders according to common underlying pathogenic processes, which from the point of view of developmental psychiatry makes a lot of sense. The DSM-5 has taken steps along this line of thinking as indicated by the most recent regrouping of disorders into the current DBD cluster. In other words, we are not defining mental disorders at discrete entities but rather along a continuum, from normal to normative, prepathological, and finally pathological disorders. Along such a spectrum, maladaptive aggression and antisocial behavior are entirely in line with developmental thinking. This way of conceptualizing psychopathology is long overdue, having gone missing in the previous versions of the descriptive diagnostic systems. It needs to be well integrated into psychiatric diagnostic classifications of children and adolescents. In short, a simple transplant of an adult model for psychiatric disorders is not realistic or helpful. We discuss the spectrum of aggression disturbances in more detail at the end of this chapter in the Clinical Implications section.

More supporting evidence for our suggestions and the developmental psychopathology view comes from neuroscience, which goes beneath the descriptive symptom level. Our field is increasingly moving away from the nineteenth-century model of strict localization of functioning toward a model that reflects the brain's seemingly endless flexibility. Recent studies have demonstrated the great interconnectivity of diverse brain areas once thought to serve distinct and exclusive functions. (Shine et al., 2016). Such interconnectivity facilitates the performance of complex tasks, such as adaptive living. This is a normal or prepathological state, which probably is related to brain development and human maturation. Under this line of thinking, the common co-occurrence of internalizing and externalizing disorders during adolescence and school age may be more a function of a heightened interconnectivity. As one brain circuit supporting antisocial or aggressive behavior becomes dysfunctional, it rapidly affects other circuits dedicated to diverse adaptive tasks, such as threat detection and risk avoidance, impulse control, and reward seeking. The preservation of isolated functioning is perhaps more quickly eroded in young developing brains, leading to a rapidly spreading dysfunction in multiple circuits. As currently configured, the DSM system (somewhat less so than the ICD system) in such cases postulates separate, distinct disorders. The developmental model looks for an underlying primary process that starts the dysfunction, as difficult as that may be, with our current state of knowledge. From the point of view of developmental psychopathology, we would see the emergence of primary, single diagnoses as a developmental and adaptive "achievement," a kind of crystallization of an adaptive—or maladaptive cluster of symptoms, as Sroufe and Rutter have suggested (Sroufe, 1997; Rutter & Sroufe, 2000; also see Figure 2.2).

Under a developmental mode, we expect that as the patient progresses in age, disorders would be more easily delineated and differentiated. By contrast, the younger the patient, the less distinct the disorders are and the more blurry the picture on a descriptive level. This thinking is applicable to other disorders such as in the differentiation into schizophrenia and bipolar disorder. Very often it is impossible to tell when the first psychotic episode occurs whether this is a predominant disorder of cognition (schizophrenia) or affect and mood (bipolar). A similar scenario can be advanced for DBDs: in the younger age ranges, the clinical picture is murky; as the patient ages and matures, his or her symptoms may fall progressively in line with specialized disordered antisocial and aggressive behavior, along the subtypes described in the proactive/instrumental/planned (PIP)/reactive/affective/defensive/impulsive (RADI) subtypes, introduced in chapter 1, discussed further and in chapter 4 on etiology.

We have practiced for many decades in the care of DBDs, and a note of clinical realism is in order: it can be difficult, if not impossible, to characterize and completely eliminate other conditions, despite all our best efforts, leaving clinicians with multiple overlapping diagnoses that also manifest with antisocial,

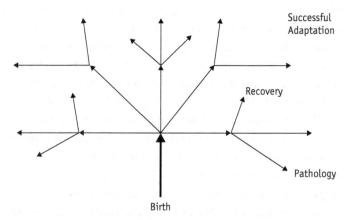

Figure 2.2 Psychopathology as an adaptive or maladaptive outcome over time. The shaping of genetic endowment by epigenetic influences. Source: Sroufe (1997).

aggressive, and even violent behavior. In such a situation, it might be best to switch to a target symptom approach in treatment, which we discuss in more detail in the Clinical Implication section in this chapter and in chapter 5 on treatment. Very often such a switch is necessary when the clinician is under considerable time pressure without access to all relevant information. DBDs often are complicated by emergencies where patients are a true danger to others and/or themselves. Then of course we do all in our power to keep everyone concerned safe and treat as best we can without a single explanatory diagnosis. Such an approach may also be extremely common in general practice, as an informal poll of practitioners indicates. At a 2016 Stanford Continuing Medical Education event we hosted about 300 attendees. During a presentation on the topic of DBDs, we asked the audience how many of them relied on the DSM or ICD for guidance when faced with a patient with some DBD. There was a small group of about 20 clinicians who raised their hands. The remainder operated along the lines of the target symptom approach.

2.2 Additional Terms Commonly Found in the Literature Related to DBDs

Antisocial behavior: behaviors that violate either laws or common rules about getting along well with others. Disobeying traffic signs, jumping a line, failing to pay bills, parking in handicapped spots, breaking the speed limit, and stealing items from stores are all good everyday examples. These are extremely common behaviors that have little or no predictive power (think of adolescent bike riders running stop signs on a daily basis on their way to school). Antisocial behaviors tend to be very prevalent in the adolescent age range, and as such they are normative, part and parcel of adolescents measuring their independence versus interdependence.

Delinquent behavior: a category and a term derived from criminology that refers to adjudicated antisocial or aggressive behavior. In this case the behavior has come to the attention of the police and the courts and has resulted in some form of punishment. This also is an extremely common occurrence, especially in youths from impoverished neighborhoods and those of an ethnic minority status. Again, isolated delinquent acts have little or no predictive power, even when the crime is sometimes of considerable gravity. In anonymous retrospective studies, young men admitted to a 30% conviction rate, mostly referring to crimes committed while adolescents. Recent statistics suggest that roughly a third of Americans have a history of arrest. (See http://www.sentencingproject.org/wp-content/uploads/2015/11/Americans-with-Criminal-Records-Poverty-and-Opportunity-Profile.pdf.)

Psychopathy: a term introduced by Hervey Cleckley (1941) in his milestone book *The Mask of Sanity*. It has been eliminated and replaced—regrettably—in the DSM system by the term *antisocial personality disorder* (APD), a construct that in our and other studies does not perform well because it is too vague and broad. The ICD system in its current iteration retains it as a special subtype. The term still survives in the criminological literature and in the newer neuroscience literature, where developmental studies increasingly support the notion that there are rare individuals (even in prison populations) who have documented disordered brain circuits serving arousal, thrill seeking, and empathy induction. This is usually regarded as the most pernicious, long-lasting, and untreatable variant of a DBD. The most infamous serial killers (such as Ted Bundy) have been assigned to this category. We discuss this very important research in some detail in chapter 4.

How do we best understand the relationship of these medical and other terms? In order to clarify how these terms are best thought of in relationship to medical terms such as DBDs we offer a schematic in Figure 2.3. We plot prevalence and persistence of these labels on the two axes of the graph. The terms themselves are presented as differently colored areas on the schema (Steiner, 2011).

As mentioned, there are two axes of relevance: prevalence, that is, how common is this problem? (plotted on the *y*-axis vertically and increasing from bottom to top) and persistence, that is, how likely is this problem to stay on and not disappear without intervention (plotted on the *x*-axis, increasing from left to right)?

Antisocial behavior is extremely common, especially in the adolescent age range. There is a rare individual that has not violated some law or another

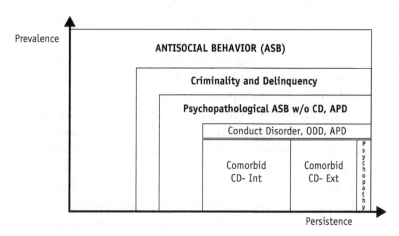

Figure 2.3 The relationship between antisocial and aggressive behavior and psychopathology.

(as mentioned, by jaywalking, talking a pencil from school, parking illegally, speeding, owning a weapon and bringing it to school, experimenting with drugs). Almost all of these behaviors go undetected and are not adjudicated. It is estimated that for each adjudicated antisocial act, there are 120 that are not known. Such antisocial age limited acts have very little predictive value, as the majority of people desist from further antisocial behavior and only a much smaller portion turns into career criminals. In fact, most of the crime committed in the adult years is attributable to a very small percentage of the population, somewhere between 7% and 11%, depending how crime is defined and what legal codex is used. The next band is defined as a band of antisocial and aggressive acts that are adjudicated but do not cluster into one of the DBD diagnoses. As we will see in our discussion in chapter 3 on epidemiology, many of these acts are not limited to DBDs but occur in the context of psychopathology other than DBDs, such as autism, attention deficit hyperactivity disorder (ADHD), bipolarity, and substance abuse disorders just to name a few. The chances that these types of behaviors persist increase in this group, especially if we are considering disorders where youth have profound problems understanding laws and rules and who are not cognizant of the wrongfulness of their acts or the laws that they are breaking because they are perhaps intellectually challenged, out of touch with reality, very excitable, or impulsive.

The final clusters in the graph show diagnosable DBDs (e.g., ODD, CD, APD). As they present with an increasing psychopathological load (i.e., as permitted by the subtypes of the ICD), they become less common. The chances of persistence begin to increase, as DBDs acquire additional problems, especially of the externalizing kind, like for instance substance abuse. And psychopathy is the smallest category in terms of prevalence but has the highest chance of long-term persistence. We are now accumulating seminal findings that have come from New Zealand that confirm this pattern over an extended period of prospective follow-up, to be discussed in some detail in chapters 3 and 6.

Figure 2.3 is intended to help the reader appreciate the importance of careful delineation of these terms, their relationships, and their importance as we prepare to effectively treat youngsters and their families. The graph also provides some justification for medicine entering the field, which for so long was dominated by criminological thinking. Juvenile justice and criminology are important areas, yet they are not able to solely address DBDs and the impact they have on society. Some years back, it was estimated that for each crime we pay a heavy price, ranging from millions when we speak of murder, hundreds of thousands of dollars (2008) for sexual assault, and thousands for vandalism and counterfeiting, not to mention human cost. In comparison to that, treatment costs pale (McCollister, French, & Fang, 2010; for further discussion, see chapters 5 and 6).

2.3 The Current Most Prevalent Taxonomies of DBDs and Their Problems: The DSM-5 and ICD-10

Taxonomy: "the systematic classification of disorders and diseases" (Stedman, 2006).

The *classification of mental disorders* is also known as psychiatric nosology or taxonomy. In psychiatry, and all medical fields, it is a key first step in any clinical or research activity. As of this date, we have two widely established systems for classifying mental disorders—the DSM-5, produced by the American Psychiatric Association, and the tenth revision of the International Classification of Diseases (ICD-10), produced by the World Health Organization.

Both systems define several categories of disorders, clustered into groupings that are believed to share many common characteristics. The clusters in both systems vary, but each disorder in the DBD cluster is thought to represent separate types or categories. Both classifications employ operational definitions, based on patient and clinician reports. Thus both systems rely extensively on subjective, not objective, symptom descriptions. These symptoms are intended to be atheoretical with regard to etiology (causation), although on closer reading one can detect a biological reductionist prejudice, implying that ultimately these symptoms will be reduced to some biological state or trait deficit or a biological marker at the very least.

The ICD system can be differentiated from the DSM by its greater emphasis on transcultural factors in the consideration of diagnostic practices in countries across the globe. This makes sense, given the charge of the World Health Association, the backer of that diagnostic system. Both the ICD and the DSM have found wide acceptance in psychiatry, as they seem to facilitate communication with colleagues and insurance companies.

As much as crisply defined categories are the desired standard in the practice of medicine, there is also a substantial scientific debate about the relative validity of a "categorical" versus a "dimensional" system of classification. Such a discussion is especially important when we approach DBDs, because, as we shall see, the current diagnostic categories have only limited validity. By adding dimensions to achieve subtypes, we could help increase the precision of these diagnoses and ultimately help practitioners in their decisions regarding a rational approach to treatment and healing. Most recently, there have been concerted efforts to converge the ICD and DSM diagnoses and their respective codes. As a result, the manuals have become much more comparable—a positive—although significant differences remain.

On the negative side, many questions of validity and utility have been raised, by scientists, ethicists, economists, and politicians. Most prominent have been concerns regarding the influence of the pharmaceutical industry, the inclusion of certain controversial diagnoses, and the stigmatizing effect of being categorized or labeled.

These concerns have led to an active pursuit of other, noncategorical efforts at defining DBDs. Usually these are more commonly encountered in psychology, especially developmental and experimental psychology, as well as in clinical psychological practice. Dimensional approaches are sometimes combined with categorical approaches to refine certain diagnoses, and if a diagnosis cannot be established, dimensions are used in targeting certain symptoms part of the presenting problems. The introduction of the age of onset as a defining characteristic in CDs or the use of the callous–emotional dimension to achieve increased accuracy of prediction are two examples for DBDs in the DSM system.

Within the dimensional approach to diagnosis, classification may instead be based on broader underlying disease spectra, arrays of normal, normative premorbid, morbid, and extreme disorders. Such an approach is an intrinsic part of a developmental perspective on disorders. As we will see as we discuss developmental aspects of these symptoms, aggression and antisocial behavior waxes and wanes in different developmental periods, being normative in one and pathological in another.

The main problem with dimensional classifications is they can be of limited value in clinical practice where yes/no decisions often need to be made, often under some time pressure, if the presentation is acute (Is this person a danger to others?), or when the practitioner has to decide whether a person requires treatment. Nevertheless, noncategorical dimensional approaches have their place in clinical psychiatry and psychology, a fact that is beginning to be discussed increasingly in medical taxonomies.

Another important criticism of both the ICD and DSM systems targets the underlying assumption that one is able to capture the nature of a disorder by relying almost exclusively on either subjective descriptions of behavior as reported by various observers, such as parents, teachers, and medical personnel, or symptoms as reported by individuals themselves, without any reference to so-called somatic information (e.g., laboratory tests, imaging studies, x-rays, just to name a few). As we discuss in chapter 4 on etiology, developmental psychiatry has reached a point where we can start rationally introducing these types of data into the definitions of DBDs. The findings from autonomic arousal across the developmental span from infancy to young adulthood and the recent findings from functional magnetic resonance imaging in psychopathic individuals show great promise.

We next turn to the most recent controversies and critiques directed mostly at the DSM system, starting with the third edition and continuing up to the most recent edition, the DSM-5. As the DSM and ICD systems evolved over the past five decades, there were many that welcomed their contributions. Their most positive aspect was that they both represented a significant move beyond random diagnostic practice or single target symptom diagnosis, as was practiced almost exclusively in the 1950s and 1960s in psychiatry. One only needs to think of how common it was to have a patient or even a nonpatient committed involuntarily to a mental health facility, as Rosenhan's (1973) study at Stanford so dramatically showed. His study used eight healthy "pseudo-patients" who presented to 12 different psychiatric hospitals in five different states. They reported as per protocol that they heard a voice. When asked what the voice said, they reported "Thud." They answered all follow-up questions truthfully. All researchers were admitted and diagnosed with psychiatric disorders. In the hospital the "patients" acted normally; however, all were forced to take antipsychotic drugs, which they mostly disposed of in innovative ways. Seven were diagnosed with schizophrenia "in remission" before their release.

It is very difficult to imagine that this crucial experiment could be done again today, as we have acquired many polithetic taxons that make such errors much less likely. Viewed this way, the DSM has grown in the aftermath of this impressive experiment. This growth has helped the profession avoid the dehumanizing consequences of psychiatric practice, silencing incisive criticisms such as those advanced by Thomas Szasz (1961).

However, very soon after the introduction of the system, another problem arose: with each new edition, the list of disorders grew. In the first DSM 106 disorders were listed. In DSM-5 we are faced with 374. Most of these currently listed disorders supposedly have a prevalence between 1% and 10%, with a mean close to 5%. Extrapolating from these numbers, this would mean that about one in five Americans (range 4% to 40%) is mentally disordered, a number that simply is not credible. Something must be wrong with the diagnostic categories, such as the process of their conceptualization, their validation, or both. As the DSM swelled from a sleek 137 pages in 1952, including all appendices, to 991 in the DSM-5, many critical voices arose. Unfortunately, DBDs are particularly vulnerable, as we shall see in our discussion throughout this chapter. Fortunately, the growth rate of the DSM categories has slowed in the transition from the fourth edition, text revision [DSM-IV-TR] to DSM-5 (e.g., the third edition had 494 pages; the fourth edition [DSM-IV]almost doubled that to 886 pages; DSM-IV-TR 943 pages; and the DSM-5 has 991). Perhaps this is the result of refining the system, which is increasingly backed by better methods and rational arguments, debated in public rather than protected by special consultant agreements.

A recent article by Widiger and Clark (2000) highlights some of the continuing problems in the DSM system. The authors contend that most of its diagnoses and criteria sets are highly debatable, and almost every sentence in the DSM can be challenged, simply because there is an absence of research guiding the construction of the DSM versions up to the DSM-IV. These critical voices led to a reconfiguration of the task force conceptualizing and testing the DSM categories, but the outcome (i.e., the DSM-5) still carries the burden of many of the same problems regarding the earlier versions. Widiger and Clark call for more transparency regarding the process of development; the clearer delineation of normal and abnormal functioning; the actually valid differentiation of diagnoses (we will see this is very relevant in our discussion when we compare ODD and disruptive mood dysregulation disorder [DSM-5 296.99, ICD-9 F34.8]); the differentiation of state and trait diagnoses (i.e., transient versus chronic problems); and stronger consideration of more objective criteria such as laboratory measures in the generation of diagnostic criteria (we will discuss this in greater detail as we consider the different etiologies for DBDs in chapter 4).

The criticisms extend to the current version of the DSM. One such powerful voice was that of Thomas Insel, the former director of the National Institute of Mental Health (NIMH). In a blog post from April 29, 2013, he writes,

> The goal of this new manual, as with all previous editions, is to provide a common language for describing psychopathology. While DSM has been described as a "Bible" for the field, it is, at best, a dictionary, creating a set of labels and defining each. The strength of each of the editions of DSM has been "reliability"—each edition has ensured that clinicians use the same terms in the same ways. The weakness is its lack of validity . . . Patients with mental disorders deserve better.
>
> —(Insel, 2013)

Subsequently, the NIMH developed an effort to create a new classification system, the research domain criteria (RDoC) for research purposes, which resulted in several sensationalist headlines. In a compromise statement, the then American Psychiatric Association president Jeffrey A. Liebermann and Insel assigned a split purpose for the two systems: DSM for clinical care and RDoC for research. It is in this spirit that we approach the current diagnoses in the DBD domain in the DSM, but we also advocate for the inclusion of recent research findings in arriving at clinical diagnoses and treatment planning. The DSM platform is a reasonable first step for the clinician. But in order to be effective in the identification and treatment of DBDs, we advocate going the extra step.

Regardless of the criticisms of the validity of the DSM approach, an even more fundamental criticism can be leveled at the theoretical basis of the entire descriptive enterprise. As mentioned, the DSM and the ICD taxonomy is based on the assumption that mental disorders can be delineated on a purely descriptive basis (i.e., by listing an atheoretical number of criteria, which ultimately should end up representing discrete disease entities). The antecedent of this approach can be found in Karl Jasper's (1963) phenomenology, although in its current use "descriptive" has moved beyond Jasper's initially intended term. Jaspers developed his "descriptive phenomenology" (by postulating the correct way to approach a patient's experience is through his or her own description, applying unbiased empathy). The DSM deviates from this original conception in that, in practice, the evaluation of a person's mental health is a blend of empathic descriptive phenomenology (signs) and empirical clinical observation (symptoms). As we will see in our further discussion, the system actually often suggests that it is listing objective symptoms when in fact it still reports subjective evaluations, albeit from the examining clinician. Is it even desirable to stay at the descriptive level at this stage of knowledge in psychiatry? We think that the field of the study of DBDs has matured sufficiently to permit clinicians to look beneath the surface of what they see.

A good example in DBDs are the strong data supporting the role of arousal, reverse conditioning, and empathy induction in the etiology of DBDs, and especially in psychopathy, as we will see. Discussing the different neuroarchitectures that are relevant for the subtypes of DBDs in chapters 4 and 6 will give us a better understanding of this point. Jensen and Hoagwood, who were both at the NIMH at the time, as early as 1997, called attention to this point (Jensen & Hoagwood, 1997). Approaching the issues of classification in the DSM system from a perspective of developmental psychopathology, the authors review the constraints of current mental disorder classification systems that rely upon descriptive symptom-based approaches. They came to the conclusion that by focusing principally on superficial descriptions of symptoms, current systems fail to address the complex nature of persons' transactions within and adaptations to difficult environments. The price we pay for purporting to be a-theoretical, the DSM (in this case the DSM-IV) misses information that helps us understand individuals' functioning—or malfunctioning across various contexts. This makes misdiagnosis likely, particularly when diagnosing in nonclinical populations. The authors conclude by advocating for the application of evolutionary theory to psychiatry and psychology, a well-known variant of developmental psychopathology. These words went unheeded as the DSM-IV-TR and the current DSM-5 edition were put together. The comments still make as much sense now as they did in 1997.

The problems besetting the DSM taxonomy discussed are not new. They have plagued the enterprise ever since its inception, drawing heavy criticism from the American Psychological Association, other interested parties, experts in mental health, and even the developers of previous versions of the system. This is not the place to recount these developments, but they are readily traceable in scientific and in popular press publications. (see articles in *The New Yorker*, the

San Francisco Chronicle, and *The Gay City News* and documentaries on MSNBC, for instance; all listed under Suggested Reading and Resources) As the leadership of the project changed from Robert Spitzer, to Allen Frances, and, in its latest iteration, to David Kupfer, secrecy regarding the development of the system persisted, despite many complaints of prominent mental health clinicians, researchers, and teachers. Frances, one of the architects of previous versions of the DSM, characterized the DSM 5 as an example of "soaring ambitions and weak methodology." DBDs, unfortunately, are one of the diagnostic groupings deeply affected by these problems.

Is there some movement to deal with these problems in a helpful fashion? A new aggregation of DBDs is introduced in the latest iteration of the DSM, with some recognition that these disorders represent a spectrum of externalizing behaviors. As Europe and the United States prepared to revise their respective taxonomies, there were cautionary comments regarding the pace of the changes but also demands for the inclusion of more basic scientific information. Möller (2008, 2009) added a warning note not to be too precipitous in the desire to include neuroscientific findings in to the criteria of the DSM and ICD systems. Möller also argued against designing an entirely new taxonomy, a point of relevance given the developments in the United States involving the RDoC and DSM described. Möller argued for a cautious inclusion of dimensional additions to the diagnostic categories that would improve the utility of the existing diagnoses in the care of a particular patient, in line with the recent demands that medicine enter a phase of individual based precision care (Möller, 2008, 2009). We are very supportive of this way of thinking.

Let us now turn to a discussion of the diagnoses in the newly formed DSM cluster of DBDs. From the point of view of developmental psychiatry, the DSM-5 is a small step in the right direction. Box 2.1 lists the cluster and their DSM and ICD codes.

Added to the DSM-5 core DBD diagnoses of CD and ODD are new DBD groupings of several other diagnoses, formerly in the DSM-IV chapter "Impulse-Control Disorders Not Otherwise Specified": kleptomania, pyromania, and intermittent explosive disorder. As we will see in chapter 3 on epidemiology, these are quite rare disorders, whose empirical support remains very weak. Another newcomer to this grouping is APD, listed here and in the chapter on personality disorders, under cluster B. ADHD has been moved to neurodevelopmental disorders. For both these changes, there is some logic, but it is not spelled out, and the empirical support for this decision is lacking. Still, this clustering approaches one possible solution to the diagnostic dilemmas we are facing in the DBD grouping: it approaches these disorders as a diagnostic spectrum that ultimately should be shown to have an underlying common dysfunctional substrate. As we will see in chapter 4 on etiology, there are several good candidates to be studied: self-regulation and impulsivity, affect and mood dysregulation, focus and distraction, aggression in its cold and hot form, and empathy and appreciation of social rules of conviviality, just to name a few.

Specific changes in the diagnoses listed under DBDs are as follows (see the relevant pages of the DSM-5 for the exact descriptions of each symptoms and their clustering algorithm).

1. Symptoms for ODD are broken down into three clusters: angry/irritable mood, argumentative/defiant behavior, and vindictiveness (here, by the way, is an excellent example for our points regarding the difficulty of creating symptoms in isolation, without referring to a specific process, history, or context. How would we know that a certain expression, feeling, or behavior is vindictive if we do not know about a description of the acts and injuries suffered by the patient?). The CD exclusion is deleted. ODD and CD can coexist. We are not told why this was changed, again. The DSM system has been going back and forth on this issue, without shedding much light on what drives this indecisiveness. We think this might be a very problematic change that could be improved if one created a dual disease spectrum that followed the PIP/RADI distinction of aggressive and antisocial behavior. On the positive side, the criteria were also changed with a note on frequency requirements and a measure of severity. These are interesting, but again it is unclear where these numeric requirements come from, how the cut points were established, and how they were tested.

The diagnostic criteria for CD, for the most part, are unchanged. This is unfortunate, as we currently have access to a great deal of new epidemiological and basic science information that could help us refine this important diagnostic category (see chapters 3 and 4). On the positive side, a new specifier was added for patients showing callous and unemotional traits on the basis of a respectable amount of published research. These traits include reduced guilt, callousness, uncaring behavior, and reduced empathy. There were some concern about the potentially stigmatizing nature of the term "callous–unemotional" so the label was changed to "with limited prosocial emotions" in DSM-5. The addition of this specifier reflects efforts to identify syndromes characterized by combinations of clinical and neurocognitive features. Callous–unemotional traits, which occur in fewer than half of young persons with CD, identify a subgroup with distinctive clinical features and neurocognitive perturbations. Patients diagnosed with CDs with callous–unemotional traits have a poorer prognosis and treatment response (see the discussion in chapter 5).

The age specifier was retained—a good decision from our point of view. Both of these specifiers have immediate diagnostic and treatment implications, as we have indicated previously and as will become clearer as we review the latest literature and discuss etiology and treatment.

2. Intermittent explosive disorder is now permitted in patients all the way down to age six. Explosive acts are no longer limited to violent aggression but can be verbal and so forth. There is a new frequency criterion and the requirement that the outburst be based in anger and cause distress and impairment, including problems with money or legal entities.

To summarize, this listing of the new DBD grouping in the DSM-5 has many face valid positive characteristics, but the exact reasons and the empirical basis for all these changes are not known nor discussed in the DSM, nor are they publicly available. There is a hint in the descriptions of these disorders that they are thought to be conceptually linked on the descriptive level. There is some discussion in the overview of the DSM DBD chapter that these disorders are characterized by problems in self-control of emotions and behavior, manifesting themselves uniquely in the violation of the right of others (through aggressive acts, even violence, and acts of vandalism and theft) and conflict with significant norms of society and authority figures (such as teachers, judges, and police). The attempt to stay at a descriptive, atheoretical level, however, strains to meet clinical and research demands, which could perhaps be better satisfied by introducing factors from neuroscience and clinical studies that lead in the direction of different causal processes.

2.4 Comparing the DSM-5 and ICD-10

The ICD-10 or DSM-5 classification on the surface seem quite similar but remain quite disparate in some respects. The assignment and grouping of the diagnoses shows this openly. The ICD-10 labels and classifies intermittent explosive disorder as "other habit and impulse disorder" and antisocial personality disorder as "dissocial personality disorder" grouped under personality disorders, among other significant differences. While the two systems, ICD-10 and DSM-5 set out to accomplish similar goals, it seems that, at times, their paths intersect for reasons that are not always clear.

Some of the differences can be attributed to the different purposes the systems are intended to serve. Historically, the ICD, established by the World Health Organization, was created in an effort to refine the diagnosis and classification of mental disorders in a way that makes diagnoses in nonindustrialized nations with impoverished resources possible. As the title describes, it is a tool that has set a variety of international standards and provided impetus for production of assessment instruments that are universally implemented. There is a much stronger emphasis on transcultural aspects of medical practice as in the DSM.

As mentioned, the ICD-10 separates DBDs into a few different categories, compared to the grouping per the DSM-5, focusing on CD and ODD alone. Within the ICD-10 ODD is classified under CD, as though it is a subtype, as indicated by the diagnostic code. CD is ascribed the number F91 while ODD is ascribed F91.3. The ICD-10 criteria description for CD maintains similar themes as described in the DSM-5 yet lists 24 separate criteria that may apply to a variety of subcategories under CD, a difference we find positive and helpful as the clinician struggles with assigning a place to many comorbid conditions.

ODD is actually defined by the ICD-10 as CD at a younger age, requiring that the CD criteria be met in order to use the diagnosis of ODD, suggesting that the two disorders are not distinct but occur on a continuum. As we mentioned, there is a rationale for this position as much as for the current DSM-5 version, which separates the two disorders again into two distinct categories. But neither system produces the necessary data to settle this issue decisively.

The ICD-10 entitles the classification as F90-F98 "behavioral and emotional disorders with onset usually occurring in childhood and adolescence." Hyperkinetic disorder remains in this grouping; the DSM has removed ADHD from it. Within the ICD-10 classification one can find the diagnoses of kleptomania, pyromania, and APD categorized under "disorders of adult personality and behavior."

The actual diagnostic criteria in both systems have been made identical. What remains different is the subtypes. Age-specific subtypes and severity ratings are identical. The DSM has introduced the callous–unemotional subtype not present in the ICD. All others are confined to the ICD. These (family context constrained, socialized versus unsocialized, depressive, hyperkinetic). The ICD-10 asks the clinician to make every effort for inclusion of a variety of symptoms within a diagnostic category. It presents it to be unfavorable to arrive at more than one diagnosis.

Three of the DBD diagnoses are classified in the ICD-10 as "other habit and impulse disorders," including intermittent explosive disorder, pathological firesetting, and pathological stealing. The DSM-5 offers fewer specifiers to guide these diagnoses, while the ICD-10 lists differential diagnostic rule outs to clarify these diagnoses.

APD, as known by the DSM-5, is captured in the ICD-10 as dissocial personality disorder, which allows a clinician to choose three of six qualifying criteria. The DSM-5 provides a greater degree of specification as it parses the diagnosis into different domains of functioning and demonstrated functional impairment for a particular criterion.

A highly instructive picture of the problems with our current grouping of DBDs emerges when we take a summarized look at what happens in the future of those diagnosed with one of them and the relationship between the diagnoses in the cluster over time. Figure 2.4 summarizes that information (Steiner, 2011; Steiner & Remsing, 2007).

Summarizing data across several studies of ODD, CD, and APD, Figure 2.4 shows that, beginning at age three to six, taking cohorts of afflicted children, after six years of prospective follow-up only 60% of the original cohort continues to be diagnosed with ODD. Treatment effects were not tracked or controlled. It was not possible from the DSM-IV array of criteria, let alone the individual symptoms, to predict positively who desisted or persisted being an ODD patient. Stability coefficients across studies ranged from .33 to .81; however, 5% of the samples provided most of the stability (68%). This is not strong support for the ODD label as configured in the DSM-IV. It is possible that the additional criteria for frequency and severity the DSM-5 offers might help in this regard, but this is an open question. Cohesive, concurrent, discriminant, and predictive analyses are needed to move beyond this problem.

A similar and equally discouraging picture emerges if we look further into the future: at age 16 to 18, only a little more than one-third of the original cohort will be diagnosed with CD; and at young adult age, around 12% will be diagnosed with APD. In both cases, as in the case of ODD, it was not possible to predict from baseline or follow up who would persist and desist. The claim is often made that this is so because ODD, CD, and APD are distinct illnesses. From a developmental standpoint, this is highly unlikely: conceptualizing these disorders as pathological derailments of normal human functioning, they appear more related than distinct. (Steiner, 2011; Steiner & Remsing, 2007) As discussed previously, the various DSM and ICD committees have gone back and forth on this issue, and the two systems treat the relationship of ODD and CD

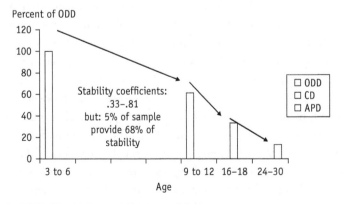

Figure 2.4 ODD, CD, APD—persistence and desistence.

in a different fashion. It is not possible to know at this point which of the options described is the best solution. From a developmental theoretical perspective, we prefer the concept that these diagnoses are related disorders and age-specific manifestations of a dysfunctional common underlying system of antisocial and aggressive behavior.

2.5 A Selective Review of the Representative Current Literature

In 2009, Olsson reviewed the criteria for CD as listed in the DSM. Primary sources were drawn from Medline, PsychInfo, and the Social Sciences Citation Index. He concludes that while the diagnostic criteria as put forth in the DSM system make it appear that patients diagnosed with CD are very much like each other, the empirical literature shows that these patients are actually quite heterogeneous (Olsson, 2009). The prevalence of more boys than girls suffering from this problem is confirmed. CD seems to describe a very stable condition the younger the patient is when the problem starts, lending more justification to the age specifier in the DSM and ICD systems. High rates of comorbidity are confirmed, just as in older studies with criteria preceding the DSM-IV classification. The author then advocates strongly for adding dimensions of other subtype classifiers, especially internalizing disorders, to do better justice to clinical realities, which ultimately must influence the prognosis and treatment. Thus the persistent problems in the DBD cluster outlined in our theoretical discussion persist, at least as far as CDs are concerned (Olsson, 2009).

A particularly informative and rare longitudinal study sheds some new light on DBDs. In 2010 David Fergusson and colleagues described the results of having followed a New Zealand birth cohort consisting of 995 youth ages 14 to 16 until they were 25 years old. This study examined potential associations between DSM-IV diagnoses of CD, ODD, and ADHD and subsequent problems in early adulthood in the realms of substance use, mental health, relationships, parenting, education, employment, and criminality. The results of this study indicated that increasing severity of DBDs and/or ADHD was associated with greater problems in early adulthood. As the severity of CD increased, so did the likelihood of early pregnancy/parenthood, substance use issues, reduced educational achievement, increased criminality (e.g., property and violent offenses), interpartner violence, and the development of APD. Youth with more severe forms of ODD were more likely to have engaged in criminal behaviors and develop internalizing problems (e.g., anxiety and depression). ADHD severity was associated with reduced levels of academic achievement and lower income. After controlling for the effects of CD, youth with ADHD did not display a significantly increased risk of criminality, substance use, or other mental health problems. Another noteworthy finding in this study was the lack of evidence indicating gender-based differences among outcomes in early adulthood for youth with CD, ODD, and ADHD. This study was important in that it showed the utility of viewing DBDs and ADHD through an additional dimensional perspective. It also supports the subclassification of DBDs along the axes of internalizing and ADHD dysfunctions, as captured in the ICD. This becomes increasingly important, as we now are fairly certain that the treatment of internalizing disorders and ADHD is quite distinct and specific. The study is unique in that the sample size and retention is large and the follow-up period extensive, crossing at least two developmental phases (Fergusson, Boden, & Horwood, 2010).

Another very positive and relatively recent development in the DBD literature is the increase in studies that include the subtyping based on callous–unemotional traits, based on a dimensional approach. This dimension has been shown to directly link to some promising neuroscience progress, which we discuss in chapter 4 on etiology.

Pardini, Stepp, Hipwell, Stouthamer-Loeber, and Loeber (2012) examined incorporation of the callous–unemotional subtype of CD in the DSM-5, specifically in relation to girls. This study used a sample of 1862 girls from Pittsburgh, Pennsylvania, between the ages of six and eight. A little over one-third of the girls in this study were in families receiving public assistance. It was hypothesized that girls with the callous–unemotional subtype of CD would engage in more severe forms of antisocial behavior and experience lesser degrees of internalizing problems (e.g., depression, anxiety). Those CD girls who did not have callous–unemotional personality traits were expected to exhibit greater internalizing problems. The authors also tracked the outcomes of girls who had callous–unemotional traits yet did not meet formal criteria for CD. This study measured the initial degree of internalizing problems, externalizing problems, academic functioning, and global impairment in girls and reexamined these areas six years later. Pardini and colleagues found that CD girls with callous–unemotional traits tended to have more severe forms of externalizing symptoms and relational aggression per parent and teacher reports than girls with CD who did not. The CD girls with callous–unemotional traits also tended to engage in more bullying behavior per teacher reports and were rated by parents and study staff as having a greater degree of global impairment when compared to girls with only CD. The girls with callous–unemotional traits that did not meet formal criteria for CD had more symptoms of ADHD and ODD than girls with neither CD nor callous–unemotional traits. They also tended to attain lower levels of academic achievement relative to controls. This study showed how the callous–unemotional subtype identified CD girls prone to less anxiety and a greater proclivity for aggression. Pardini and colleagues' work also demonstrates callous–unemotional traits as predictors for future problems regardless of whether a young girl has ever met formal criteria for CD (Pardini et al., 2012). The finding raises the question as to whether callous–unemotional traits are an early marker for the development of certain subtypes of DBD. It begs the question: Should we concentrate on callous–unemotional traits as a dimension, perhaps type (psychopathy, for instance) to gain better positive predictive power? In our discussions of "hot" versus "cold" types of conduct problems, we elaborate on the pros and cons of such an approach.

In 2015, the term *callous–unemotional traits* took on fresh nomenclature in Randall Salekin's review article, in which he noted the addition of the "with limited prosocial emotions" specifier to the diagnosis of CD in the DSM-5. We believe that this addition has been a step in the right direction in trying to identify youths with DBD who might be headed for the worst possible prognosis. We previously observed the challenge DSM-IV criteria for DBDs encountered to identify youth who manifest psychopathic traits in young adulthood, a very important question. Salekin advocates that additional dimensions of childhood psychopathy, namely grandiose–manipulative and daring–impulsive traits, should be incorporated into the diagnostic classification of CD. While callous–unemotional traits are an important component of childhood psychopathy, Salekin argues that it is difficult to maintain these are core features of psychopathy, given their relative scarcity of empirical validation (Salekin, 2016). Furthermore, available literature suggests that, like callous–unemotional traits, grandiose–manipulative and daring–impulsive traits are identifiable in youth and relatively stable over time. This is an interesting argument, as it links the callous–unemotional characteristics to an interpersonal dimension of psychopathy that forms part of the Hare checklist approach to psychopaths and certainly fits the clinical and forensic descriptions of such individuals. We pursue this discussion further in chapter 4 on etiology and chapter 6 on forensics.

Salekin (2016) cites evidence illustrating the correlation of grandiose–manipulative and daring–impulsive traits with specific such as "ringleader bullying," substance use, diminished school performance, accident propensity, and aggressive behavior. He discusses extant research suggesting that young people with psychopathic personality traits tend to have differing cognitive and emotional profiles than that of their nonpsychopathic CD peers and that this may be moderated, at least in part, by the dimensions of psychopathy that predominate in an individual. Salekin also describes how current research suggests that biological correlates of childhood psychopathy often vary according to the predominating set of psychopathic traits. In one such example, low heart rate has been most highly correlated with youth possessing daring–impulsive traits and, to a lesser yet still significant degree, grandiose–manipulative traits. However, youth with predominating callous–unemotional traits do not tend to have reduced heart rates as compared to peers who lack psychopathic traits. Salekin concludes that before we expand the specifiers for CD in a manner that better identifies youth with psychopathic traits, further research is needed to better understand how these proposed specifiers relate to CD youth (Salekin, 2016).

Yet another very positive recent development in the DBD diagnostic literature is the increasing influence of neuroscience and research diagnostic criteria on this important domain of psychopathology. Blair, Leibenluft, and Pine's (2014) review article published in *The New England Journal of Medicine* summarizes both the clinical and neurocognitive aspects of CD and associated callous–unemotional traits, lending a great deal of weight to this form of subtyping. Youth with callous–unemotional traits tend to have a reduced response to distressing situations. It is postulated that this is the result of deficiencies in empathy. For instance, these youth often do not respond to distressing situations (i.e., emotionally and/or physiologically) in a typical manner and frequently do not recognize when others are frightened or upset. At the neurocognitive level, young people with callous–unemotional traits tend to have a reduced amygdala response to distressing situations. However, anxious and traumatized youth with CD who lack callous–unemotional traits tend to have an elevated amygdala response to fear-inducing situations, overestimate potential threats in their environment, and as a result are more prone to reactive aggression. (Blair et al., 2014) Once again, the ICD subtypification into CD with and without internalizing disorders receives considerable support. As mentioned and further discussed in chapter 5, these findings and concepts have major implications for the treatment of CD youths.

Support for these important distinctions also comes from another group of researchers. In their 2008 review article, Frick and White highlight that youth with callous–unemotional traits make up a distinct subgroup of the youth characterized as antisocial and/or aggressive. They are prone to more severe forms of aggression that frequently persist throughout the youth's developmental maturation. Evidently, this severe aggression is further qualified by emotional, personality, and cognitive differences when compared to antisocial youth who lack callous–unemotional traits. Frick and White added characterization with reference to two additional subgroups commonly seen in youth with psychopathic traits: "arrogant and deceitful interpersonal style" and "impulsive and irresponsible behavioral style." This widely cited review article marked an important step forward in articulating the need to better identify youth, particularly at risk for aggressive and antisocial behavior (Frick & White, 2008).

Some researchers have even gone as far as investigating the notion that callous–unemotional traits may represent a "psychiatric diagnosis" in their own right. A 2012 review article by Herpers, Rommelse, Bons, Buitelaar, and

Scheepers examines this possibility. Despite a need for more studies to determine whether callous–unemotional traits represent a distinct diagnosis or personality type, this review suggests that callous–unemotional traits, in general, are identifiable, relatively stable over time, and predict more severe conduct problems (Herpers et al., 2012). While further study would be helpful, via extensive review in 2014, Frick, Ray, Thornton, and Kahn support that, at the very least, a thorough clear understanding of callous–unemotional traits can inform the diagnosis and treatment of youth who have severe CD.

The DSM-5 focuses almost exclusively on behaviors when classifying individuals with DBDs minimally differentiating the aggression profiles, temperaments, and personality traits observed among youth with DBDs. For this, we look to the pioneering work of Hervey Cleckley, Robert Hare, and an ever-growing body of research, summarized in the aforementioned review by Frick and colleagues (2014). A minority of individuals with well-established patterns of antisocial behavior have psychopathic or callous–unemotional traits, setting the stage for engagement in extreme forms of antisocial behavior and violence. Psychopathy as a construct seems to produce increasing evidence that this might be a relatively homogenous group with distinct deficits in functioning at all levels: biological, psychological, and social.

Frick and colleagues (2014) cite research of genetic background, early attachment style, and adverse childhood experiences playing a role in the development of individuals with callous–unemotional or psychopathic traits. These individuals tend to be less responsive to the emotional states of others (e.g., they display poor recognition of fear or sadness in others) and display a dampened biological reactivity to stressful situations (e.g., reduced variability in heart rate and diminished galvanic skin response). They also possess a cognitive style that makes them relatively indifferent to negative reinforcement and fail to utilize empathizing with others as a means for navigating social interactions (Frick et al., 2014).

The available research on CD youth with psychopathic or callous–unemotional traits suggests that a conglomeration of the factors outlined can result in scenarios leading ultimately to most pernicious outcomes: individuals who lack concern for the welfare of others; recklessly pursue their desires; are calm in the face of brutality; and see violence, manipulation, and/or deceit as a tool for having their own personal needs met.

A review by Kahn, Frick, Youngstrom, Findling, and Youngstrom (2012) published in the *Journal of Child Psychology and Psychiatry*, highlights the developmental psychopathology perspective as an important framework for enhancing our field's understanding of DBDs. Frick and colleagues outline three important factors that a developmental approach to psychopathology plays in furthering our understanding of severe conduct problems.

1. Developmental approaches to understanding psychopathology prioritize how developmental trajectories deviate from the norm in children with severe behavior problems instead of merely summarizing their known risk factors (e.g., In what ways do harsh parenting practices negatively impact a youngster's ability to self soothe?).

2. A developmental psychopathology perspective rejects the idea of a "cookie-cutter" or "one-size-fits-all" approach to understanding children's conduct problems. That is, there are a number of ways that a young person's developmental trajectory can be derailed, thus leading to a poor outcome. In essence, a developmental psychopathology approach looks at risk factors in relation to the developmental pathways they intersect.

3. Frick and colleagues describe development as an ever-changing, "dynamic and ongoing process." Thus youth with severe conduct problems do not represent "static" biologically predetermined diagnoses. Rather, they are akin to moving targets whose trajectories are influenced by a variety of factors. For example, a DSM-5 diagnosis provides us with a way of categorizing a certain type of outcome (e.g., CD), yet tells us nothing about the developmental processes that went awry leading to such an outcome (e.g., poor abilities to self-soothe, impulsivity, and/or deficits in the ability to empathize with others).

4. A developmental psychopathology approach acknowledges that people are capable of, and often do, change with time. In order to best characterize and treat behavior problems, we need to be aware of the factors that impact their stability over time. Furthermore, it is not absolute that the factors that contributed to a given "outcome" (e.g., a diagnosis of CD) in a young person will be the same ones that predict its stability, or lack thereof, over time.

Frick and colleagues go on to provide a description of how the development of callous–unemotional traits in youth is largely influenced by problems in the development of conscience. Central to the development of conscience is one's capacity for empathy and guilt. Youth with callous–unemotional traits do not readily experience either. Frick and colleagues succinctly describe the emergence of callous–unemotional traits in youth essentially as wayward conscience development (Kahn et al., 2012).

We can bring these complex findings from research more to life if we include an example from the humanities. Let us consider two characters from popular culture who both seem to have met criteria for a diagnosis of CD. First, we consider Matt Damon's character from the film *Good Will Hunting*. Will Hunting is an exceptionally bright, talented, and severely traumatized young man, prone to bouts of reactive aggression. Now consider the main character from Stanley Kubrick's film *A Clockwork Orange*, Alex DeLarge, who was played masterfully by Malcom McDowell. Alex is a crafty 15-year-old boy with a reduced capacity for empathy who terrorizes others for sport. Both of these youth could easily be labeled as having CD. However, these are two vastly different individuals whose treatment and prognosis in a "real-world" scenario would be quite different. In their review article, Blair and colleagues (2014) rightly point out that CD youth with callous–unemotional traits have distinct clinical and neurocognitive profiles, tend to be less responsive to intervention, and ultimately have a less favorable long-term prognosis.

Despite our grim characterization of youth and adults with callous–unemotional traits, there is good reason to believe that our growing understanding of this condition will lead to better identification and individualized treatment approaches. Frick and colleagues (2014) reference two approaches that have shown promise in treating youth with callous–unemotional traits: parent training interventions and multisystemic therapy. Both of these approaches are detailed in the Chapter Five.

Interestingly, children with a "fearless" or what is sometimes referred to as "behaviorally uninhibited" temperament tend to develop conscience less readily than others. These fearless children are those daredevils who will explore previously uncharted territory (e.g., climbing a rickety bookshelf, going down a tall slide head first) with little concern about potential punishment. They also tend to not be intimidated, experience less anxiety, and are less physiologically aroused by unfamiliar people or situations than peers. Frick and colleagues go on to summarize how parenting practices have been shown to influence the development of conscience in children with a fearless temperament.

Research elucidating the match or mismatch between a child's temperament and parenting styles is astute and noteworthy. It is our opinion, based on research findings and clinical experience, that parenting practices and a variety of other early life experiences can play a major role in determining whether these "fearless" children go on to become prosocial risk-taking individuals (e.g., firefighters, helicopter rescue pilots, world-class rock climbers) or antisocial adults with a facility for violence. For this reason, it is imperative that we consider a young persons' temperament, personality, and aggression profile when assessing youth for DBDs and formulating treatment plans.

Hubbard, McAuliffe, Morrow, and Romano (2010) describe the ways that reactive and proactive aggression are the result of differing developmental trajectories and are associated with different behavioral outcomes. They also provide an excellent summary of the questionnaires used to assess for reactive versus proactive aggression. While many of the described questionnaires show validity error, a 36-item questionnaire developed by Little, Brauner, Jones, Nock, and Hawley (2003) has shown great promise in characterizing the adolescent aggression profile.

A review by Viding, Fontaine, and McCrory (2012) outlines the differences in antisocial behavior among youth with callous–unemotional traits and those who lack such traits. Youth with callous–unemotional traits appear to have a genetic predisposition to engage in aggressive, antisocial behavior. In contrast, the antisocial acts of youth and lack of callous–unemotional traits seem to be primarily influenced by their environment (e.g., poor parenting practices). Although it was not the focus of this chapter, we contend that the discussion of the impact a youth's environment has on antisocial behavior underscores the reasons why socioeconomically underserved and ethnic minority youth are overrepresented within the United States' juvenile justice system. Children who grow up in environments with endemic financial, educational, and social barriers are going to be exposed to more risk factors with the potential to negatively impact their developmental trajectories. These findings essentially confirm the original Hans Eysenk hypotheses regarding the origin of conduct problems in two major pathways, which explained the adverse outcomes as an interaction between individual characteristics (arousal) and context (criminogenic versus noncriminogenic environments). Eysenk's work was carried forward by Adrian Raine and others, adding support to the hypothesis as follows: high arousal (anxious children) rapidly orient toward their social context and environment. When raised in a criminogenic setting, they will turn antisocial very rapidly; by contrast, low arousal (low anxious or perhaps callous–unemotional) children will resist any social contextual influence. They will turn out antisocial in any environment, especially in those that actively reinforce and model antisocial behavior and aggression as positive behaviors and desirable characteristics.

2.6 Implications for Clinical Practice

Currently we have available to us practice parameters regarding the major disorders in the DBD grouping in the US, continental Europe and Britain. All of these, in varying detail, discuss the special obstacles and difficulties the clinician encounters in the assessment of externalizing disorders, where we usually have patients resistant to and intimidated by the clinical process, coupled with the potential danger of punishment by either parents, school or the judicial authorities.

(National Collaborating Centre for Mental Health & Institute for Social Care, 2013; Steiner, 1997; Steiner & Remsing, 2007). The existing practice parameters are essentially in agreement on the major points regarding clinical practice and DBDs (National Collaborating Centre for Mental Health & Institute for Social Care, 2013).

Currently, there are no practice parameters for intermittent explosive disorder, kleptomania, pyromania, and APD published by the major organizations for psychiatry and child and adolescent psychiatry in the United States.

As is needed with all patients, we start by succinctly describing one's profession, role, and purpose for interview. Sensitive points are those that have brought the individual to treatment, a possible legal breech, strongly negative feelings of parents or primary caregivers, or the denial of the patient him- or herself who may be unable to identify as the patient. Here we discuss the almost inevitable difficulties the clinician encounters and the diagnostic process. These problems go beyond what we usually encounter in the treatment of adolescents. They are particular to externalizing disorder, such as DBDs (Steiner & Hall, 2015).

The foundation of the clinical interview is the working alliance, as in other disorders, but even more so with patients in this grouping. The establishment of quick rapport with the subject being interviewed is of course always a goal but may not be easily attainable in the first session. The goal is rapid increase of comfort level, combined with a large download of pointed, directed information regarding symptoms and severity, which sometimes are not consensual. Very often patients will feel unjustly accused and worried about the consequences of their actions. This is easily understood when we review the list of symptoms we are interested in, which essentially are transgressions against family, rules, and maybe even laws. The most useful clinician stance early on has to be one of dispassionate inquiry, as hard as that may be to achieve and maintain, given the nature of some of the symptoms we are about to hear described. A useful attitude is one of "let me hear from you what sort of problems people are saying you are having" while not guaranteeing any confidentiality, as we may well discover imminent danger to self or others, which is so common in these patients.

As this process is taking place, consideration needs to be given to the context of the antisocial and aggressive acts. For example, a boy who lives in the midst of significant community of gang violence and is often targeted when he walks down the street could be understood to be living in a different context of violence when he repeatedly gets into fights with members of other gangs in the neighborhood. In contrast we might see the context of violence differently around a young girl who is engaged in significant social and physical violence along with her friends against a new girl in the high school.

If we find ourselves needing more information, this is most easily accomplished by interviewing caregivers separately, including school personnel and police and juvenile justice employees, ideally before we meet the patient for the first time. The assessment of CD includes information obtained directly from the child as well as from the parents regarding the core symptoms of CD, age of onset, duration of symptoms, and degree of functional impairment. But it also good to remember that studies have shown that parents, teachers, and even police often do not know the full extent of externalizing antisocial and aggressive behaviors—some estimates go as high as 120 event per symptom known about. Siblings or concerned friends might be less compromised informants, always provided the patient agrees to have them included in the clinical process.

Usually, youth with CD often have had multiple contacts with schools, police, and other agencies. Beyond parents, school officials and teachers are often the first people to note behavioral changes or emerging CD patterns. Schools are the context within which truancy, changes in grades, association with problematic peers, or atypical behavioral patterns tend to emerge. Often schools are the initiating point of referral for the mental health clinician. Given the amount of time that youth spent there, schools are also well positioned to work collaboratively as part of the treatment team when parents give consent for such contact.

Any degree of police or court involvement should be taken seriously because of the relatively high threshold required to prompt action from these authorities. Many of the symptomatic behaviors that define CD can easily lead to police or official involvement. Clinicians need to be aware that most police officers and courts have limited training in mental health issues and even more limited training in the specifics of child and adolescent mental health. The collaborating clinician can use these situations as opportunities to share experience and information about youth psychiatric disorders. While specific communication about a particular youth will be informative, having ongoing collaborative relationships with police and courts can make interventions more effective. Where specialized mental health courts are available, clinicians might consider making appropriate referral to such authorities.

It also is important not to rule out the necessity for repeat contacts, should the situation remain obscure, nor do we expect to fully comprehend a case after a single session. That would be the exception, not the rule. Often we are left with missing decisive information to arrive at a firm DBD diagnosis. As we would expect, this is more common the older and more "crime-seasoned" a patient becomes. In these circumstances, it is useful to remind the patient that we are clinicians, not police officers, and that our job is to diagnose, not judge. Our role as to be helpful to the patient, first and foremost. This may enable us to gather the necessary information to arrive at a diagnosis.

Still, having given talks in many clinical and academic settings, we are aware that many clinicians dealing with DBDs do not use the descriptive diagnostic system at all, except for insurance purposes, where its helpfulness is also often limited because reimbursement is limited. There are also colleagues that use the systems in very idiosyncratic ways, especially as far as the DBDs are concerned. When asked why this is so, the usual reply is: applying these diagnostic labels is not very useful, and it does not lead to a particular intervention or set of interventions that promise to give good results. These clinicians rely on their clinical experience almost exclusively, which of course can be vast and helpful but also significantly skewed. A similar situation exists in forensic psychiatry, as we discuss in chapter 6. It looks like this problem has come to the attention of the architects of the DSM diagnostic systems, judging by some recent publications on how to remedy the situation.

A group of authors set out to discuss several options regarding improving the utility of the DSM system for clinical practice. These options are not based on any empirical information of how clinicians actually are using the system. The authors call for a systematic study of this issue as a starting point (First & Westen, 2007). As we commented, in one of our larger audiences at Stanford in 2016, there was only a small minority of attendees who professed to employ the DSM as they were trying to diagnose DBDs. Another suggestion is to introduce a standardized severity dimension across all diagnostic categories. The five-axis system in the previous iterations of the DSM, which was dropped for this revision, somewhat served this purpose. The Global Assessment of Functioning scale had limited usefulness because of its confused conceptualization of anchoring points. The other suggestion is to evolve a prototype matching system that is close to a clinician's thinking. This seems like a very complex task and very difficult to empirically test, establish, and earn, as many of the diagnoses in the DBD grouping are quite far removed from prototypes. More to the point, they are too general to be helpful. The way we would suggest is based on a comparison that Thienemann, Hamilton, and Hamilton (2007) proposed.

Thienemann et al. (2007) sees the best use of the DSM system and structured interviews as a broad platform that diligently combs through all possible symptoms to make sure that the clinician does not overlook any problems. We would support such a conceptualization as well. The DSM is a start to establish a clinical base. But one needs to go beyond it, in the case of DBDs, to arrive at a useful position.

In addition to the interview, we suggest the use of standardized screening instruments (symptom scales and possibly structured interviews, which can provide a depersonalized way of gathering vital information and complementing the clinical exam and the behavioral reports by school, guidance personnel, and police reports; Huemer, 2012). A few that involve excellent psychometrics are the Conners' Parent Rating Scale, the Youth Self Report, the Child Behavior Checklist, the Barratt Aggressive Acts Questionnaire, and the Conners/Wells Adolescent Self-Report of Symptoms (Steiner & Remsing, 2007).

The widely used Child Behavior Checklist and Youth Self-Report as developed by Achenbach and colleagues provides a clinically useful screening instrument (Achenbach, 2011). These scales enable broad screening for both internalizing and externalizing symptoms and provide DSM-oriented diagnostic clusters and relevant T-scores. What is especially useful in this tool is that aggressive behaviors are outlined on one subscale and diagnostic likelihood is reported for both ODD and CD patterns based on DSM criteria. We have used the aggression subscale in several studies to delineate hot aggression. The delinquency subscale was used to measure cold aggression. Both of these scales produced credible, important results with high schoolers and incarcerated delinquents, both populations with high ecological validity. Other scales are available and are listed in Table 2.3.

These scales are important and help us reach some more definitive conclusions. But, like any laboratory test in medicine, their use is auxiliary to the clinical interview and the descriptive diagnosis. Ideally the results of these scales are available prior to the clinical interview or are produced in an intervall between the first and second session. We let youths complete these scales on their own, while meeting with parents regarding development, marital status, and issues and summary of school performance. Most patients—even those in custodial settings—are remarkably open in their answers to these instruments, as we have found in our studies in the California Youth Authority. The neutral setting of completing a report in a quiet room seems to reduce the defensiveness in the

Table 2.3 **Commonly Used Instruments to Measure Antisocial Behavior and Aggression**

Scale	Abbreviation
Anchored Brief Psychiatric Rating Scale	BPRS–C-9
Brief Psychiatric Rating Scale—Children	BPRS-C
Child Behavior Checklist	CBCL
Youth Self Report	YSR
Child Behavior Rating Form	–
Children's Aggression Scale—Parent Version	CAS-P
Children's Global Assessment Scale	C-GAS
Modified Overt Aggression Scale	M-OAS
Pediatric Inpatient Behavior Scale	PIBS
Severity and Acuity of Psychiatric Illness Scales	SAPIS

Note: For a more complete listing see Steiner and Remsing (2007).

Sources: Achenbach (2011); Halperin, McKay, & Newcorn (2002); Jaspers (1963); Knoedler (1989); Kronenberger, Carter, & Thomas (2003); Lachar et al. (2001); Lyons (1998); Overall & Pfefferbaum (1982); Shaffer et al. (1983); Steiner & Remsing (2007).

patient, if the scale is properly explained and set up, and the results can later be used to provide a focal point for discussion of complex issues.

We next describe in detail the steps in the entire assessment process that promise to lead us to fruitful conclusions with DBD patients. We also illustrate each step with specific case examples. Overall, the goal is to arrive at a primary or at least principal diagnosis—see our list of definitions (are we dealing with a DBD, rather than ADHD, for instance?). Furthermore, one should attempt to assign the presenting problems to a primary or secondary disorder (are the reported drug sales part of a antisocial repertoire that is reinforced by peers or even parents [CD], or are they driven by cravings and the need to supply one-self with substances [substance abuse disorder]?). If all else fails, then we suggest a preliminary target symptom approach while the necessary information is gathered to determine the principal or primary diagnosis (How do I stop this patient from carrying out the threat against his school? Does he have the means to perpetrate a shooting?)

The *first step* in the assessment, following the proper introductions and setting of the examination is obtaining as a detailed as possible description of the antisocial-aggressive event that triggered the referral. If there are many, we usually focus on the most recent or most significant one. In the case of a forensic referral, these events are usually described by the charges brought against the patient or outlined by the lawyers involved in the case (more on this in chapter 6). A hallmark of this first examination of an event is the determination of the context in which the acts occurred. Connor's (2012) description of maladaptive aggression best illustrates the characteristics that should raise the clinician's suspicion that psychopathology of yet undetermined nature is at the bottom of the event in question. He provides an excellent framework to help us see that in a particular event, antisocial behavior and aggression has lost their adaptive purpose and function.

1. *Aggression that occurs independent of an expectable social context.*

Example: During a scout meeting a child walks over to the scout leader and punches him in the face. The topic discussed was about the long history of scouting.

2. *Aggression that occurs in the absence of expectable antecedent social cues.*

Example: An adolescent on a bus walks over to another passenger reading a newspaper, grabs the paper, tears it up, throws it to the ground and calls the passenger, an elderly gentleman whom he has never seen before, a series of highly insulting names.

3. *Aggression that is disproportionate to its causes in intensity, frequency, duration, or severity.*

Example: A boy is told by his parents that he must stop playing video games and start his homework. In response, he throws the game console through the living room picture window and breaks the television screen. He then proceeds to bash in his mother's car's windows with a crow bar.

4. *Aggression that does not terminate after apologies have been offered.*

Example: A girl keeps verbally attacking another girl who inadvertently stepped in front of her in the cafeteria line, even after she apologizes and lines up behind the accuser. She continues to call her highly insulting names and accuses her of "disrespecting" her and having eyes for her boyfriend. The two girls are not friends or even acquaintances and attend different grades.

If the clinician obtains any descriptions like the ones listed, this should raise a suspicion that there might be a psychiatric reason for the patient's action. The next question to be answered is whether this was an isolated act or there have been several in the past few months. If we obtain a history of many of such events, be they either similar or diverse, that should lead to a more careful and comprehensive psychiatric assessment to see whether the patient actually meets diagnostic criteria set forth by our current taxonomic systems.

The *second step* in our clinical asessment consists of going through the entire list of symptoms listed in the DBD grouping to arrive at a primary diagnosis. Since ADHD, learning problems, substance abuse and dependence, depression, and posttraumatic stress disorder (PTSD), just to name a few, have been found to be so extraordinarily prevalent in this population, special attention should be given to the symptoms of these disorders, while making an attempt to ascertain that these are either partial syndromes or developmentally start after the onset of the DBD in question.

If we are certain that there are indeed two or more diagnoses present, we then will assign a primary disorder and a secondary disorder. (e.g., a youth with severe CD who is part of a gang and thus gets exposed repeatedly to traumatogenic events, resulting in PTSD). The clinician would first target the CD symptoms to disrupt the repeated exposure to trauma. Such a sequence also makes sense from the point of view of compliance with treatment: it is highly unlikely that an active gang member would stick to a PTSD protocol while continuing being active part of a gang.

It is of course also possible that, from a devlopmental point of view, the patient was an innocent bystander in a gang-related incident, resulting in PTSD. Subsequently, he develops increasing problems with academic performance, sleep, affect regulation, and impulsivity under stress. This leads to his truancy from school, trying to avoid task demands that he cannot meet or peer contacts who are threatening reminders of the event. In such a case, the patient might meet CD criteria, but the first concern would be to control the PTSD symptoms to re-establish sleep, attention, ability to perform on tests, and compliance with school demands.

Another sequence we encounter very frequently is the co-occurrence of substance use, abuse, and even dependence with CD symptoms. It is usually crucial to determine what came first: casual drug experimentation, leading to abuse and possibly dependence, which in turn is supported by antisocial and aggressive behavior, such as stealing, selling drugs, prostitution, intimidation of others with weapons, and stealing and robbery. Substance abuse could be the primary diagnosis that needs to be treated in order to control CD symptoms. Box 2.2 gives a summary of diagnoses that should always be considered in the diagnoses and treatment of DBDs, based on many comorbidity data (discussed further in chapter 3 on epidemiology).

In working with this population of DBDs, it is very often the case that the clinician is in a position where he or she does not have all the necessary information in hand to decide which course of action to take. The situation is worse when there is great time pressure to decide, as is so often the case with DBDs where danger to others and to self is almost always a realistic concern. The refined developmental approach may simply not be possible. In such a situation, clinicians usually switch to a *target symptom approach,* where the control of the most dangerous and destructive symptom becomes the focus of clinical intervention. With this approach, we are buying time to gather information that is missing while protecting others and the patient from harm. It is less important to be specific but more important to be effective and quick. As we will see in the treatment chapter, the

---

Box 2.2 **Primary Disorders of Aggression Other than DBDs That Are Commonly Associated with Antisocial and Aggressive Behavior**

ADHD, combined type

Substance use disorder

Anxiety disorders

Mood disorders

Pervasive developmental disorder, autism

Mental retardation

Schizophrenia, especially paranoid type

acute treatment of DBDs employs all possible biopsychosocial interventions to stabilize the patient. And, as we will see in chapter 5, there is enough information in the literature for a more refined psychopharmacology that is informed by the third step to be described, the classifying of antisocial and aggressive acts into hot and cold ones. Table 2.4 summarizes the distinctions between the diagnosis-specific primary disorder versus the target symptom approach.

The *third step* in our assessment of antisocial acts and aggression aims to establish a better characterization of the symptoms in the light of the most recent and relevant neuroscience findings. Target symptoms can be divided into two important subcategories, which have important implications for cause, treatment, and prognosis in clincial as well as in forensic practice (for the latter see chapter 6). Having started this discussion in chapter 1, we next add some more details to deepen the reader's understanding of where current neuroscience, clinical consensus, and research lead us.

Antisocial and aggressive acts constituting DBD core symptoms can be of two basic varieties: emotionally charged (hot) or planned in cold blood (cold). In leading the Stanford/Howard/AACAP workgroup in this discussion, we had our 50 some participants discuss and define such a bipartite distiction. The group consisted of roughly equal parts of researchers, practitioners, and academics with a special background in DBDs. The results of these discussions were reviewed by several international experts of DBDs, whose feedback helped us refine the proposed subdivision.

Table 2.4 **Connection of Primary Disorders to Target Symptom Approaches**

Primary Disorder	*Target Symptom Approach*
Primary disorder (curative intent)—diagnostic types (CD, ODD, etc.)	Target symptom (palliative intent)—relevant dimensions (i.e., callous–unemotional, aggression, delinquent behavior, etc.)
Diagnosable disorder	Significant problem in the context of insufficient data, time pressure, complex presentation
No extensive comorbidity	Extensive comorbidity
Typical symptom presentation	Atypical symptom presentation
Sufficient information from clinical trials about specifically efficient treatments (e.g., GABA enhancers, mood stabilizers, stimulants)	Nonspecific treatments, broadband interventions (e.g., antipsychotics)

Note: CD = conduct disorder; ODD = oppositional defiant disorder.

Table 2.5 summarizes the various antecedent models for this proposed distinction, which have been studied over several decades in criminology and sociology, psychology, and psychiatry. Most of the authors mentioned in this table have a long and distinguished track record of researching and publishing similar bipartite and sometimes tripartite systems. The relevant labels specific to each author are indicated on the table as bold, with neutral or less relevant labels in regular print.

These polarities can be easily compared and lead one to see intuitively the commonalities underlying these labels. The work group then agreed to create new composite labels to catch the essence of these distinctions in the aggregate.

1. *PIP:* antisocial acts and aggression are those that are carried out with malice and forethought. These acts are often covert, hidden from public view, disguised, and disavowed. The individual perpetrating them is cooly planning these acts, which are meant to enrich, acquire, diminish the other person involved, and perhaps wreak revenge upon others. The accompanying emotional state is perhaps a positive one: one anticipates a good outcome—more territory, a meal, an so on. The best animal model for PIP is the cat lying in wait for the mouse to appear. The cat is quiet, focused, calm, determined to strike when possible. The anticipated outcome is positive. The act is seen in a positive light without regret; the perpetrator feels justified in the use of this social instrument. The neuroscientific platform that supports this behavior is extensive, drawing on all possible brain resources in the service of bringing

Table 2.5 **Antisocial and Aggression Subtypes and Their Theorists**

Empirically Supported Antisocial Behavior and Aggression Subtypes	Researcher or Theorist
Overt/Oppositional Covert	R. Loeber (Loeber & Schmaling, 1985)
Reactive/Proactive	K. Dodge (Dodge, 1988)
Affective/Predatory	B. Vitiello (Vitiello, Behar, Hunt, Stoff, & Ricciuti, 1990)
Defensive/Offensive	R. J. Blanchard (Blanchard, Hori, Tom, & Caroline Blanchard, 1988)
Socialized and Undersocialized	H.C. Quay (Quay, 1993)
Impulsive/Controlled	E. Magargee (Megargee, 1966)
Hostile/Instrumental	M. Atkins & D. Stoff (Atkins & Stoff, 1993)
Impulsive/Premeditated/Medical	E. Baratt (Barratt, Monahan, & Steadman, 1994)

this act to a successful conclusion. (We discuss further details of this point in chapter 4 on etiology.)

2. RADI: antisocial acts and aggression. These acts are negatively emotionally charged. They usually accompanied by or triggered by anger, sadness, and fear. They are unplanned and impulsive. They are overt—easily witnessed. There are few if any attempts to disgiuse the act. Perpetrators are usually aware that they have transgressed; they feel bad about the act and often apologize. They take repsonsibility for these behaviors and feel ashamed or guilty. The perpetrator connotes these acts as negative, hurtful, and not right and anticipates that the outcome of these acts will have negative consequences. RADI is supported by a completely different neuroscientific platform: RADI is part of the threat detection system and is triggered in a dose-responsive fashion (again, more of this in chapter 4 on etiology). If the perpetrator feels greatly endangered and sees little or no escape, that will lead to an RADI act. The animal model closest to this form of antisocial behavior or aggression is the sleeping cat who does not anticipate that its tail is going to be stepped on, who then turns around, makes itself as big as possible, and hisses and growls, looking maximally excited, angry, and scared. The classic human example would be the child suffering physical abuse at the hand of the parent, who attacks with little warning and whom the child cannot leave because they are too young and dependent to do so.

Evidence from neurobiology and psychology of aggression supports these two major phenotypes of aggressive behavior. RADI or hot aggression is an emotionally charged form that often is poorly thought out and highly reactive to situational stimuli; this form of aggression is known to have links to serotonin, dopamine, norepinephrine, and GABA systems and to be rooted in the neuronal architecture of the limbic system (an activation locus) and the prefrontal cortex (a controlling and shaping locus). RADI aggression is by far the more common form of aggression and is seen in multiple contexts.

In passing, we want to mention that all legal codices known to date have acknowledged—implicitly or explicitly—this distinction. A crime committed with malice and forethought versus one committed in the heat of passion is usually labeled differently (murder vs. manslaughter) and punished differently, with the codices usually allowing more leeway for the RADI variety (more on this in chapter 6 onforensic implications).

From a clinical standpoint, this distinction has immediate implications for treatment: because PIP acts are supported by a wide range of brain ciruitry distributed over the entire cortex, as is usually the case with instrumental behavior, it should basically be unresponsive to interventions that are limited in their range of therapeutic mechanisms. Thus medication(s), especially narrowband medicines such as SSRIs, perform not particularily well. Broadband medicines such as gabaergic enhancers might have more of an impact. To put it provocatively, short of rendering the patient unconscious—or physically containing him or her—we cannot expect much impact on PIP. RADI, by contrast, should be much more responsive to medications and interventions that reduce negative emotionality, threat perception, and impulsivity. As we will see in chapter 5, this can be achieved by several different forms of biopsychosocial interventions.

So far, the treatment outcome literature has not utilized the distinctions we have made here. Treating samples of patients with DBD diagnoses where such a heterogenity is not controlled would lead to, and indeed does lead to, weak or even absent treatment effects. These have been the rule in many treatment outcome studies as discussed in chapter 5 (also see Lipsey & Wilson, 1998). Our workgroup has called attention to this problem and suggested concrete solutions to move the field in a more positive direction (Connor et al., 2006).

Some of these arguments were resumed by many of the members of our workgroup with the Food and Drug Administration as we were seeking to obtain an indication for the treatment of hot aggression specifically, but these efforts led to only modest progress (Jensen et al., 2007). Feedback from the agency indicated that the current diagnostic categies in the DBD cluster were not seen as valid enough to grant such an indication. An argument to make a parallel decision to the indications for "pain" or "fever" (i.e., specific target symptoms instead of diagnoses) produced only very little support from the agency. Regrettably, in the absence of a specific indication for the treatment of any of the symptoms or syndromes of DBD, it is very unlikely that we will see major investments into clinical studies that would improve our databases and knowledge regarding efficiency and efficacy of the treatment of DBDs.

The *last step* in our assessment is the physical and laboratory exam. In our practice we expect that a pediatric or adolescent medicine exam and pertinent laboratory tests are on file that are not older than six months. This is necessary because the literature has repeatedly and credibly reported that there are multiple potential medical sources of DBD symptoms. Prospective data from population-based studies have shown that any chronic pediatric illness is more likely to result in externalizing behaviors and potential disruptive patterns (Cadman, Boyle, & Offord, 1988; Cadman, Boyle, Szatmari, & Offord, 1987; McDougall et al., 2004). Central nervous system injury and neurological disorders are especially common and can originate from a variety of diseases. Lead poisoning or other heavy metals can result in neurological problems, which then display with behavioral dysregulation. In addition, malnutrition and disorders of metabolism can also in rare instances produce effects on the body that result in disruptive patterns. Finally, chronic and neurological illnesses of various types can make children feel poorly and produce outward symptoms of disruptive behaviors, which are driven by their internal sensation of illness. Children often lack a framework to understand the somatic processes in their bodies and may instead present with behavioral manifestations. Dorothy Otnow Lewis and her colleagues have, over the past 20 years, documented an astounding degree of comorbidity between violence, aggression, and neuropsychiatric injury in forensic populations. She has found that a large proportion of severely aggressive offenders have traumatic brain injuries, severe mental retardation, and epilepsy. In aggregate, these central nervous system insults may have roots in the significant degree of childhood violence and abuse that many extreme offenders have been subject to at developmentally critical periods (Lewis, 1983; Lewis & Pincus, 1989; Lewis et al., 1988; Yeager & Lewis, 2000). This is obviously pertinent for a comprehensive assessment, especially in forensic populations. We resume discussion of this topic in chapter 6 on forensics.

We do not, as a matter of routine, perform physical exams ourselves in this population. One reason for this is that many times the patients are victims of physical and sexual abuse, which calls for the highest level of caution and sensitivity. This is best left to a well-equipped primary care office. Second, the types of physical problems that could be relevant are usually way beyond the scope of psychiatric practice and are best left for our medical colleagues to pursue. We do, however, recommend that at the very least a height, weight, body mass index, and set of standardized vital signs at rest are made part of the psychiatric assessment. This not only gives us general health indicators that have immediate relevance for our psychopharmacological interventions but also gives us some indication of biological risk factors for DBDs. We discuss this more extensively in chapter 4 on etiology, when we turn our attention to the connection between arousal and risk taking as well as psychopathy.

In conclusion, we would like to briefly discuss another possible solution to the diagnostic dilemmas embedded in the current DBD cluster. This proposed developmental model is based on the idea that antisocial acts and aggression occur on a continuum ranging from normal, adaptive behaviors to extremely malignant and penicious types of diagnoses. The suggested model is built on the PIP–RADI distinction discussed but preserves a diagnostic/typogical approach at the extremes of these two dimensions. As seen in Figure 2.5, we begin by establishing two spectra, which are divided by the neuroscientific platforms and descriptive characteristics discussed. The model assumes that either cold or hot acts can be present at different rates in different developmental stages. If deviating from normative frequencies during these developmental phases, these deviations would be labeled maladaptive acts. Such acts would then call for a more concered effort to arrive at a descriptive DSM or ICD diagnosis. Reshaping the current diagnostic criteria of CD and ODD to more fully comply with descriptions of PIP and RADI acts would result in CD becoming a juvenile syndromal disorder of PIP

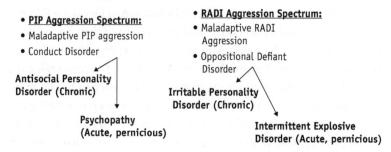

Figure 2.5 Proposed spectra of disorders of antisocial and aggressive behavior.

and oppositional disorder of RADI. If these disorders persist into adulthood, we could see two possible outcomes in each spectrum—one of a more chronic and the other one of a more acute variety. In the case of PIP, we see antisocial personality disorder as a chronic syndrome of predominantly PIP acts; the most malignant variant of that would then be the reintroduced label of psychopathy, an unrelenting, especially virulent manifestation of PIP. In the RADI spectrum, the bifurcation would be a newly created "irritable personality disorder," reflecting the chronic lower grade variant and paralleling the antisocial personality in the PIP diagnostic spectrum, and a more acute variety of RADI, labeled intermittent explosive disorder, after that existing label has been improved and tested.

Most likely, there also would be mixed or undifferentiated disorders, where the predominance of cold versus hot disturbances is not possible. From a developmental point of view, such mixed presentation would be more common in young patients or in individuals that have struggled with these problems for a long time, have not received adequte treatment, and perhaps perisist in criminogenic environments where both these dimensions of antisocial and aggressive behaviors retain some adaptive value. Such spectra would provide a more realistic diagnostic mirror for the two forms of empirically supported forms of antisocial acts and aggression. The labels hold the promise to lead the clinican to a more specific and realistic set of interventions, based on the form of antisocial acts and aggression, age of onset, and duration of illness. Needless to say, such radical changes in our taxonomic thinking would need much continued high-quality research and clincial practice. But from our perspective, it would provide an excellent pathway into the future.

References

Achenbach, T. M. (2011). Child Behavior Checklist. In J. S. Kreutzer, J. DeLuca, & B. Caplan (Eds.), *Encyclopedia of clinical neuropsychology* (pp. 546–552). New York: Springer New York.

Atkins, M. S., & Stoff, D. M. (1993). Instrumental and hostile aggression in childhood disruptive behavior disorders. *Journal of Abnormal Child Psychology, 21*(2), 165–178.

Barratt, E. S., Monahan, J., & Steadman, H. (1994). Impulsiveness and aggression. *Violence and Mental Disorder: Developments in Risk Assessment, 10,* 61–79.

Blair, R. J. R., Leibenluft, E., & Pine, D. S. (2014). Conduct disorder and callous–unemotional traits in youth. *The New England Journal of Medicine, 2014*(371), 2207–2216.

Blanchard, R. J., Hori, K., Tom, P., & Caroline Blanchard, D. (1988). Social dominance and individual aggressiveness. *Aggressive Behavior, 14*(3), 195–203.

Cadman, D., Boyle, M., & Offord, D. R. (1988). The Ontario Child Health Study: Social adjustment and mental health of siblings of children with chronic health problems. *Journal of Developmental & Behavioral Pediatrics, 9*(3), 117–121.

Cadman, D., Boyle, M., Szatmari, P., & Offord, D. R. (1987). Chronic illness, disability, and mental and social well-being: Findings of the Ontario Child Health Study. *Pediatrics, 79*(5), 805–813.

Cleckley, H. (1941). *The mask of sanity: An attempt to reinterpret the so-called psychopathic personality.* St. Louis, MO: Mobsy.

Connor, D., Carlson, G., Chang, K., Daniolos, P., Ferziger, R., Findling, R., . . . Plattner, B. (2006). Stanford/Howard/AACAP Workgroup on Juvenile Impulsivity and Aggression: Juvenile maladaptive aggression: a review of prevention, treatment, and service configuration and a proposed research agenda. *Journal of Clinical Psychiatry, 67*(5), 808–820.

Connor, D. F. (2012). *Aggression and antisocial behavior in children and adolescents: Research and treatment.* New York: Guilford Press.

Dodge, K. A. (1988, June). The structure and function of reactive and proactive aggression. Paper presented at the Earlscourt Symposium on Childhood Aggression, Toronto.

Fergusson, D. M., Boden, J. M., & Horwood, L. J. (2010). Classification of behavior disorders in adolescence: Scaling methods, predictive validity, and gender differences. *Journal of Abnormal Psychology, 119*(4), 699–712.

First, M. B., & Westen, D. (2007). Classification for clinical practice: How to make ICD and DSM better able to serve clinicians. *International Review of Psychiatry, 19*(5), 473–481.

Frick, P. J., Ray, J. V., Thornton, L. C., & Kahn, R. E. (2014). Annual research review: A developmental psychopathology approach to understanding callous-unemotional traits in children and adolescents with serious conduct problems. *Journal of Child Psychology and Psychiatry, 55*(6), 532–548.

Frick, P. J., & White, S. F. (2008). Research review: The importance of callous-unemotional traits for developmental models of aggressive and antisocial behavior. *Journal of Child Psychology and Psychiatry, 49*(4), 359–375.

Halperin, J. M., McKay, K. E., & Newcorn, J. H. (2002). Development, reliability, and validity of the Children's Aggression Scale–Parent version. *Journal of the American Academy of Child & Adolescent Psychiatry, 41*(3), 245–252.

Herpers, P. C., Rommelse, N. N., Bons, D. M., Buitelaar, J. K., & Scheepers, F. E. (2012). Callous–unemotional traits as a cross-disorders construct. *Social Psychiatry and Psychiatric Epidemiology, 47*(12), 2045–2064.

Hubbard, J. A., McAuliffe, M. D., Morrow, M. T., & Romano, L. J. (2010). Reactive and proactive aggression in childhood and adolescence: Precursors, outcomes, processes, experiences, and measurement. *Journal of Personality, 78*(1), 95–118.

Huemer, J., Hall, R., & Steiner, H. (2012). Developmental approaches to the diagnosis and treatment of eating disorders. In J. Lock (Ed.), *Oxford handbook of child and adolescent eating disorders: Developmental perspectives*: Oxford: Oxford University Press.

Insel, T. (2013, April 29). Director's blog: Transforming diagnosis. http://www/nimh.nih.gov/about/director/2013/transforming-diagnosis.shtmlJaspers, K. (1963). *General psychopathology.* Manchester, UK: Manchester University Press.

Jensen, P. S., & Hoagwood, K. (1997). The book of names: DSM-IV in context. *Development and Psychopathology, 9*(2), 231–249.

Jensen, P. S., Youngstrom, E. A., Steiner, H., Findling, R. L., Meyer, R. E., Malone, R. P., . . . Blair, J. (2007). Consensus report on impulsive aggression as a symptom across diagnostic categories in child psychiatry: Implications for medication studies. *Journal of the American Academy of Child & Adolescent Psychiatry, 46*(3), 309–322.

Kahn, R. E., Frick, P. J., Youngstrom, E., Findling, R. L., & Youngstrom, J. K. (2012). The effects of including a callous–unemotional specifier for the diagnosis of conduct disorder. *Journal of Child Psychology and Psychiatry, 53*(3), 271–282.

Knoedler, D. W. (1989). The Modified Overt Aggression Scale. *The American Journal of Psychiatry, 146*(8), 1081–1082.

Kronenberger, W., Carter, B., & Thomas, D. (2003). Pediatric inpatient behavior scale. In S. Naar-King, D. A. Ellis, & M. A. Frey (Eds.), *Assessing children's well-being: a handbook of measures* (pp. 57–62). Mahwah, NJ: Lawrence Erlbaum.

Lachar, D., Randle, S. L., Harper, R. A., Scott-Gurnell, K. C., Lewis, K. R., Santos, C. W., . . . Morgan, S. T. (2001). The Brief Psychiatric Rating Scale for Children (BPRS-C): Validity and reliability of an anchored version. *Journal of the American Academy of Child & Adolescent Psychiatry, 40*(3), 333–340.

Lewis, D. O. (1983). Neuropsychiatric vulnerabilities and violent juvenile delinquency. *Psychiatric Clinics of North America, 6*(4), 707–714.

Lewis, D. O., & Pincus, J. H. (1989). Epilepsy and violence: Evidence for a neuropsychotic-aggressive syndrome. *Journal of Neuropsychiatry and Clinical Neuroscience, 1*(4), 413–418.

Lewis, D. O., Pincus, J. H., Bard, B., Richardson, E., Prichep, L. S., Feldman, M., & Yeager, C. (1988). Neuropsychiatric, psychoeducational, and family characteristics of 14 juveniles condemned to death in the United States. *The American Journal of Psychiatry, 145*(5), 584–589.

Lipsey, M. W., & Wilson, D. B. (1998). *Effective intervention for serious juvenile offenders: a synthesis of research.* Thousand Oaks, CA: SAGE.

Little, T. D., Brauner, J., Jones, S. M., Nock, M. K., & Hawley, P. H. (2003). Rethinking aggression: A typological examination of the functions of aggression. *Merrill-Palmer Quarterly, 49*(3), 343–369.

Loeber, R., & Schmaling, K. B. (1985). Empirical evidence for overt and covert patterns of antisocial conduct problems: A metaanalysis. *Journal of Abnormal Child Psychology, 13*(2), 337–353.

Lyons, J. S. (1998). *The Severity and Acuity of Psychiatric Illness Scales: An outcomes-management and decision-support system: Child and adolescent version: Manual:* San Antonio, TX: Psychological Corporation.

McCollister, K. E., French, M. T., & Fang, H. (2010). The cost of crime to society: New crime-specific estimates for policy and program evaluation. *Drug and Alcohol Dependence, 108*(1), 98–109.

McDougall, J., King, G., de Wit, D. J., Miller, L. T., Hong, S., Offord, D. R., . . . Meyer, K. (2004). Chronic physical health conditions and disability among Canadian school-aged children: a national profile. *Disability and Rehabilitation, 26*(1), 35–45.

Megargee, E. I. (1966). Undercontrolled and overcontrolled personality types in extreme antisocial aggression. *Psychological Monographs: General and Applied, 80*(3), 1–29.

Möller, H.-J. (2008). The forthcoming revision of the diagnostic and classificatory system: Perspectives based on the European psychiatric tradition. *European Archives of Psychiatry and Clinical Neuroscience, 258*(5), 7–17.

Möller, H. J. (2009). Development of DSM-V and ICD-11: Tendencies and potential of new classifications in psychiatry at the current state of knowledge. *Psychiatry and Clinical Neurosciences, 63*(5), 595–612.

National Collaborating Centre for Mental Health, & Institute for Social Care. (2013). *National Institute for Health and Care Excellence: Clinical guidelines: Antisocial behaviour and conduct disorders in children and young people: Recognition, intervention and management.* Leicester, UK: British Psychological Society.

Olsson, M. (2009). DSM diagnosis of conduct disorder (CD)—A review. *Nordic Journal of Psychiatry, 63*(2), 102–112.

Overall, J., & Pfefferbaum, B. (1982). The Brief Psychiatric Rating Scale for Children. *Psychopharmacology Bulletin, 18*(2), 10–16.

Pardini, D., Stepp, S., Hipwell, A., Stouthamer-Loeber, M., & Loeber, R. (2012). The clinical utility of the proposed DSM-5 callous-unemotional subtype of conduct disorder in young girls. *Journal of the American Academy of Child & Adolescent Psychiatry, 51*(1), 62–73.

Quay, H. C. (1993). The psychobiology of undersocialized aggressive conduct disorder: A theoretical perspective. *Development and Psychopathology, 5*(1–2), 165–180.

Rosenhan, D. L. (1973). On being sane in insane places. *Science, 179*(4070), 250–258. doi:10.1126/science.179.4070.250

Rutter, M., & Sroufe, L. (2000). Developmental psychopathology: Concepts and challenges. *Development and Psychopathology, 12*(3), 265–296.

Salekin, R. T. (2016). Psychopathy in childhood: Toward better informing the DSM–5 and ICD-11 conduct disorder specifiers. *Personality Disorders, 7*(2), 180–189.

Shaffer, D., Gould, M. S., Brasic, J., Ambrosini, P., Fisher, P., Bird, H., & Aluwahlia, S. (1983). A Children's Global Assessment Scale (CGAS). *Archives of General Psychiatry, 40*(11), 1228–1231.

Shine, J. M., Bissett, P. G., Bell, P. T., Koyejo, O., Balsters, J. H., Gorgolewski, K. J., . . . Poldrack, R. A. (2016). The dynamics of functional brain networks: Integrated network states during cognitive task performance. *Neuron, 92*(2), 544–554.

Sroufe, L. A. (1997). Psychopathology as an outcome of development. *Development and Psychopathology, 9*(2), 251–268. doi:10.1017/S0954579497002046Stedman, T. L. (2006). *Stedman's medical dictionary.* Baltimore: Lippincott Williams & Wilkins.

Steiner, H. (1997). Practice parameters for the assessment and treatment of children and adolescents with conduct disorder. *Journal of the American Academy of Child & Adolescent Psychiatry, 36*(10), 122S–139S.

Steiner, H. (2011). *Handbook of developmental psychiatry.* Londonn: World Scientific.

Steiner, H., & Hall, R. E. (2015). *Treating adolescents.* Hoboken, NJ: John Wiley.

Steiner, H., & Remsing, L. (2007). Practice parameter for the assessment and treatment of children and adolescents with oppositional defiant disorder. *Journal of the American Academy of Child & Adolescent Psychiatry, 46*(1), 126–141.

Steiner, H., Saxena, K., & Chang, K. (2004). The psychopharmacological treatment of primary and secondary disorders of aggression. *Child and Adolescent Psychopharmacology News, 9*(7), 1–5.

Szasz, T. (1961). *The myth of mental illness.* New York: Harper & Row.

Taylor, F. K. (1967). The role of phenomenology in psychiatry. *The British Journal of Psychiatry, 113*(500), 765–770.

Thienemann, M., Hamilton, J. D., & Hamilton, J. D. (2007). Learning evidence-based practices for anxious children. *Journal of the American Academy of Child & Adolescent Psychiatry, 46*(10), 1367–1374.

Viding, E., Fontaine, N. M., & McCrory, E. J. (2012). Antisocial behaviour in children with and without callous-unemotional traits. *Journal of the Royal Society of Medicine, 105*(5), 195–200.

Vitiello, B., Behar, D., Hunt, J., Stoff, D., & Ricciuti, A. (1990). Subtyping aggression in children and adolescents. *Journal of Neuropsychiatry and Clinical Neurosciences, 2*(2), 189–192.

Widiger, T. A., & Clark, L. A. (2000). Toward DSM-V and the classification of psychopathology. *Psychological Bulletin, 126*(6), 946–963.

Yeager, C. A., & Lewis, D. O. (2000). Mental illness, neuropsychologic deficits, child abuse, and violence. *Child and Adolescent Psychiatry Clinics in North America, 9*(4), 793–813.

Suggested Reading and Resources

Carey, B. (2008, December 17). Psychiatrists revising the book of human troubles. *The New York Times,* p. A1.

Carey, B. (2012, May 9). Psychiatry manual drafters back down on diagnoses. *The New York Times,* p. 12.

Chibbaro, L. (2008, May 30). Activists alarmed over APA: Head of psychiatry panel favors "change" therapy for some trans teens. *Washington Blade.*

Cosgrove, L., & Bursztajn, H. J. (2009). Toward credible conflict of interest policies in clinical psychiatry. *Psychiatric Times, 26*(1), 40–41.

Cosgrove, L., & Krimsky, S. (2012). A comparison of DSM-IV and DSM-5 panel members' financial associations with industry: a pernicious problem persists. *PLoS Medicine, 9*(3), e1001190.

Cosgrove, L., Krimsky, S., Vijayaraghavan, M., & Schneider, L. (2006). Financial ties between DSM-IV panel members and the pharmaceutical industry. *Psychotherapy and Psychosomatics, 75*(3), 154–160.

Demazeux, S., & Singy, P. (2015). *The DSM-5 in perspective: Philosophical reflections on the psychiatric Babel.* Dordrecht: Springer.

Frances, A. (2009). A warning sign on the road to DSM-V: Beware of its unintended consequences. *Psychiatric Times, 26*(8), 1–4.

Frances, A., & Schatzberg, A. (2010, February 10). Psychiatrists propose revisions to diagnosis manual. *PBS.* http://www.pbs.org/newshour/bb/health-jan-june10-mentalillness_02-10/

Jabr, F. (2013). Beyond symptoms. *Scientific American, 308*(5), 17.

Laskowska, M. (2016). Illiterate psychiatric diagnoses and their implications for the justice system. https://papers.ssrn.com/sol3/papers.cfm?abstract_id=2808702

Owen, G., & Harland, R. (2007). Editor's introduction: Theme issue on phenomenology and psychiatry for the 21st Century. Taking phenomenology seriously. *Schizophrenia Bulletin, 33*(1), 105.

Spiegel, A. (2005). The dictionary of disorder. *New Yorker, 80*(41), 56–63.

Steiner, H., Medic, S., Plattner, B., Blair, J., & Haapanen, R. (2006). Predicting PIP and RADI aggression in incarcerated juvenile delinquents: Trama, affect and defensiveness. Paper presented at the Annual Meeting of the American Academy of Child and Adolescent Psychiatry. San Diego, October 24–29.

3

Epidemiology of Disruptive
Behavior Disorders

3.1 Definitions

Epidemiology: "the investigation and application of trends, distribution and causation pertinent to particular groups or populations with regards to health care or specific events" (Stedman, 2006).

The application of epidemiology provides information regarding incidence (i.e., number of new diagnoses within a given period of time), prevalence (i.e., proportion of new diagnoses relative to the total population), and relative risk (i.e., probability of an illness occurring among a group exposed to a disease risk factor versus a group who has not been exposed), all of which further our understanding of patterns of disease.

Epidemiological studies usually employ a variety of measures to capture risk factors for disease or disease itself. Such instruments have at least two very important properties that allow one to come to important conclusions.

Sensitivity: "in clinical pathology and medical screening, sensitivity is the proportion of affected patients who give a positive test result for the disease that the test is intended to reveal" (Stedman, 2006). A "sensitive" diagnostic tool is one in which the overwhelming majority of individuals who do not have a condition will not screen positive. Thus a positive sensitive screen does not indicate the presence of a given condition but raises the suspicion that one might be present. A positive screen helps to narrow down a list of likely candidates, conceptually similar to a police station lineup.

Specificity: "in clinical pathology and medical screening, specificity is the proportion of those tested with negative test results for the disease that the test is intended to reveal" (Stedman, 2006). This term is used to describe how we go about confirming whether an illness or mental disorder is in fact present. A diagnostic tool or algorithm that has high specificity confirms that someone who screened positive for a condition, more than likely, has said condition. Most assessments are either highly sensitive or highly specific, depending on the desired entity. At first pass, epidemiological studies cast a wide net to make sure that there are no false negatives. The closer one moves toward actual clinical practice, the more certain one should be that a disorder is in fact present and requires treatment. Such reassurance comes from highly specific instruments and procedures, such as structured interviews and objective laboratory tests.

There are more concepts in epidemiology that help us drill down into large data sets, but we limit our discussion to those aforementioned, as they have the most relevance for practicing clinicians.

The ideal epidemiological studies would start with a randomly selected sample from an entire population, employ a highly sensitive screen, and then hone in on the high and low risk portions of the sample. Increasingly detailed and specific instruments are used to establish the fact that high and low scorers indeed can be separated by fulfilling diagnostic criteria for the disease in question. Ideally, a longitudinal arm would follow, establishing, through the same process, stability of the findings over extended periods of time and the number of new cases that emerge in a given time period. Data is typically reported in reference to yearly occurrences.

In the study of disruptive behavior disorders (DBDs), one could envision the use of a screen like the Behavior Assessment System for Children—Second Edition (BASC-2), followed by the use of a battery of more specific instruments measuring aggression and antisocial behavior (listed in chapter 2) and culminating in a structured and clinical interview, capturing as many of the known biological, psychological, and social factors we know to contribute to the etiology of DBDs. As will become clear later on, the field lacks the ideal studies at the present time, but compared to previous decades, there are a great deal more studies that approach our ideal and give us confidence to speak with some authority about how frequently DBDS occur in the general and clinical populations; in part, this is another way to validate the diagnostic criteria discussed.

3.2 Discussion of the Current Literature

The following will subsections will address our understanding of the current literature. Highlighted below are developmental directions regarding the diagnoses, and statistical underpinnings of the diagnoses. One final possible pathway of the diagnoses is explored to better understand the application of the current literature.

3.2.1 DEVELOPMENTAL TRAJECTORIES OF ANTISOCIAL BEHAVIOR AND AGGRESSION

As noted in chapters 1 and 2, antisocial, aggressive, and even violent behavior are normative processes in childhood. According to *Stedman's Medical Dictionary*, normative is defined as "pertaining to the normal or usual" (Stedman, 2006). For our purposes, the normative definition may expand to encompass the understanding that a diagnosis or behavior occurs at a certain age and can still be disruptive, yet contrast with, not interfere with, normal function. Normal delineates an individual from a pathological group, whereas normative concedes that, at a certain age, certain behaviors and thoughts are so common it is hard to assign them pathological status. If, let us say, normal toddlers emit aggressive behavior every few minutes, that makes it difficult to call all toddlers pathological. We have to look at the impact a behavior has on day-to-day functioning and continued progressive growth instead.

In an important developmental study, The National Institute of Child Health and Human Development (NICHD) Early Child Care Research Network found that physical aggression, which started relatively high at age two, gradually decreased over the course of early development kindergarten and then grades 1 to 3 in elementary school (Figure 3.1). The study employed parental reports on the Child Behavior Checklist, tracking 1,100 diverse children.

Prominent predictors of the physical aggression decrease included high family resources and more sensitive parenting. Those cases demonstrating persistent aggression predicted poorer social and academic outcomes (NICHD Early Child Care Research Network & Arsenio, 2004).

This early developmental time period appears to be developmentally sensitive. The NICHD Early Child Care Network, in a recent work, found that despite parenting being, by far, the strongest predictor of childhood behavior, early negative child-care experiences could have a stressful effect on children

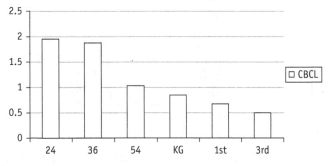

Figure 3.1 Physical aggression by parent report (CBCL) from 2 years to 8 years.
Source: NICHD Early Child Care Research Network, 69(4), Serial # 278, 2005.

that often results in elevated levels of aggression at later ages (Belsky et al., 2007). These findings illustrate one largely normative epidemiological pattern of childhood aggression. Further studies like this are needed, extending the age range and the types of antisocial behavior and aggression, as well as their deterioration into clinical syndromes. Our research group also used the Youth Self Report (YSR), regrouped the aggression items according to our model of reactive/affective/defensive/impulsive (RADI) and proactive/instrumental/planned (PIP) subtypes and compared 1,483 high schoolers and 948 incarcerated delinquents (Steiner et al., 2011). Figure 3.2 demonstrates the outcome of this research confirming our hypotheses that delinquents have significantly greater measures of RADI and PIP aggression. Hot and cold aggression, as conceptualized, particularly in chapters 1 and 2, validly separate normal adolescents from adolescents who have a better than 90% frequency of a DBD diagnosis (Niranjan S Karnik et al., 2008).

We should now attempt to broaden our understanding of these subtypes of aggression as they probably unfold across infancy to late adolescence. Taken in the aggregate, antisocial and aggressive behavior declines from infancy to early adulthood. This seems to be a general socialization effect. However, the trajectories of "hot" and "cold" aggression most likely have very different nonlinear trajectories, which need to be studied much further. Here we would like to offer a quick reminder of the distinction between hot and cold aggression, which transcends the diagnostic categories in the DBD grouping. It is always useful to differentiate what type of antisocial behavior and aggression one is witnessing: proactive versus reactive. Recall that proactive aggression (PIP) can be associated with cold, planned, thought-out aggressive acts. Perpetrators have plenty

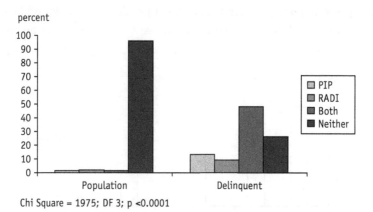

Chi Square = 1975; DF 3; p <0.0001

Figure 3.2 Comparing Clinically significant (top 2%) RADI and PIP Problems in high school students and incarcerated adolescents by expert rated YSR Aggression (RADI) and Delinquency (PIP) items (Steiner et al., 2005).

of time to mull and contemplate the acts, leading to a likely positive emotional state as they provide justification and fantasize about the expected vengeful outcome.

Meanwhile, the reactive impulsive (RADI) individual expresses a negative emotion, with little time or thought put into what may have triggered the aggression. These individuals impulsively and overtly respond within a situation. We explicate the differing underlying neuroscientific platforms for these two forms of aggression in chapter 4 on etiology.

As best as we can tell from our own research and our clinical experience in clinical and juvenile justice populations, PIP aggression does really not come online until late preschool, as it by definition requires extensive deception and planning. This requires extensive frontal lobe and more widely distributed brain resources that are not available until the age of four to six or perhaps even later. The school years see a gradual increase in PIP and a peak in early adolescence. From then on, PIP seems to decline but most likely never completely disappears, because it does have highly adaptive value when employed in a rational and considerate manner. By contrast, RADI seems to have a high peak in early infancy, declining steadily during the school-age years. The cited NICHD study reports on "overt" aggression, which most likely is equivalent with RADI—hot acts committed without much further thought. As a part of the threat detection system, RADI is most likely hard-wired form birth on or shortly thereafter. It also responds to parenting and socialization, but we would anticipate that internal (i.e., hormonal) and external (i.e., traumatic events) factors could have strong facilitating or inhibiting influences. Thus there is most likely a natural peak of RADI in early adolescence, but then we would see a gradual decline over time, similar to the decline of PIP, unless of course the person suffers from certain forms of psychopathology, such as posttraumatic stress disorder (PTSD) and/or there is a high adaptive value to being impulsively threatening such as is the case in certain pernicious environments, such as prisons. These considerations help us refine our expectations as to what we will encounter as we meet individuals from different phases of development.

3.2.2 THE PREVALENCE OF THE CURRENT DBD DIAGNOSES

We now turn our attention to what is known regarding the prevalence of the current DBD diagnoses in use (see Table 3.1). We need to retain criteria from the fourth edition, text revision of the *Diagnostic and Statistical Manual of Mental Disorders* (DSM-IV-TR) because many of the studies of the epidemiology of DBDs date several years back and report their findings by those criteria. When the fifth edition (DSM-V) cites these numbers, it is not always clearly stated

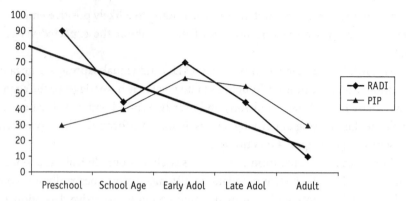

Figure 3.3 Developmental trajectories of aggression subtypes (schematic).

whether this refers to DSM-IV-TR or DSM-V criteria, which, although very similar, do contain some significant changes. In general, it can be expected—as in previous shifts between DSM iterations—that the newer criteria will result in reduced numbers, as the criteria increase and some become more stringent. Thus we currently are not entirely certain of these prevalence numbers, as the wide ranges reported indicate.

As we can tell from Table 3.1, at the present time we are still lacking crucial basic epidemiological information, especially regarding the new additions to the DBD grouping. The ranges reported in the DSMs, where they are known,—although we are uncertain as to exact source of these numbers—are still quite wide, making one question the validity of the averages reported. Summarizing these averages across diagnoses, we can assume that DBDs have a prevalence of somewhere between 10% and 16% without us knowing what exact contributions the rarer syndromes (pyromania, kleptomania, etc.) will make. Further examination of oppositional defiant disorder (ODD) reveals significant prevalence variability ranging from 1.5% to 15.5% of the population with expected greater prevalence in males, albeit inconsistent. Once introduced as a diagnosis in the third edition of the DSM in 1980, ODD prevalence has been found to vary depending on the criteria that have been used. This accounts for the observed 25% drop in prevalence between 1980 and 1987. The reasons for this observed discrepant prevalence are many and are most notably likely related to age effects, socioeconomic status effects, and the persistent problems with ODD as a polithetic taxon (i.e., a group of very diverse criteria or unknown but probably varying validity) that ultimately leads to inherent heterogeneity. ODD prevalence becomes most critical when relating to conduct disorder (CD) prevalence in that 40% of children with a diagnosis of ODD develop CD later in life. Another way of viewing links between the two diagnoses is understanding the 90% of adolescents with CD had an ODD diagnosis at some point, further demonstrating a

Table 3.1 **Prevalence Rates of DBDs**

Diagnosis	DSM-IV-TR	DSM-V
DBD	No data provided	NA
Conduct disorder	1%–10%	2%–10% with average of 4%
Oppositional defiant disorder	2%–16%	1%–11% with average of 3.3%
Intermittent explosive disorder	Rare; data is lacking	2.7%
Antisocial personality disorder	1%–3% (community samples) 3%–30% (clinical samples)	0.2%–3.3%
Pyromania	Rare; no statistics provided in DSM-IV	3.3% (sample of persons reaching criminal system with repeated fire setting
Kleptomania	5% in identified shoplifters; unknown in general population	0.3%–0.6%
Other specified disruptive, impulse-control, and control disorder	NA	NA
Unspecified disruptive, impulse-control, and conduct disorder	NA	NA

Note: DSM-IV prevalence is expected to be synonymous with DSM-IV-TR prevalence since DSM-IV-TR is only text revisions. Also, as is common for DSM, it is difficult to identify the source of these numbers. DBDs = disruptive behavior disorders; DSM-IV = *Diagnostic and Statistical Manual of Mental Disorders* (fourth edition); DSM-IV-TR = *Diagnostic and Statistical Manual of Mental Disorders* (fourth edition, text revision); DSM-5 = *Diagnostic and Statistical Manual of Mental Disorders* (fifth edition); NA = not applicable

Sources: American Psychiatric Association (2000), Steiner (2011), Steiner & Hall (2015).

low problematic positive predictive power. In other words, as we look forward from ODD in time, we cannot tell who is going to persist in the pathological trajectory, which takes the problems with antisocial and aggressive behavior outside of the family; this is one of the main distinctions between these two diagnoses. Looking backward in time, we can see how almost all the children with CD earlier had ODD. Such a continuity does suggest that our diagnostic grouping should retain the view that these two diagnoses are on a developmental continuum (as the International Classification of Diseases [ICD] is still assuming, along with the view of developmental psychopathology), while the lack of predictive power may be used to argue that these two disorders are distinct. This remains an important issue to be resolved in future studies.

Data regarding the epidemiology of CD is fairly consistent among Western countries. Maughan, Rowe, Messer, Goodman, and Meltzer (2004) retrospectively examined a survey of over 10,000 British boys and girls between the ages of 5 and 15. As has been the case with similar studies, CD was much more likely to occur in boys. Rates of CD in boys increased in a linear fashion with increasing age up to 15 years. Aggression, namely fighting, in boys with CD decreased with age. However, status violations (i.e., truancy, running away, staying out too late) increased with age.

Maughan and colleagues (2004) observed that the risk of girls developing CD remained relatively low and constant, until entering their early teens when the risk was found to significantly increase. Not surprisingly, girls with CD tended to display core symptoms like aggression to a lesser degree than boys; however, when they reached the 13 to 15 age range, girls were found to be just as prone as boys were to commission of nonviolent behaviors associated with CD (e.g., status offenses). Like similar surveys, ODD appeared to be more common in boys, but this data is somewhat equivocal. In general, the rates of ODD in youth drop significantly in late childhood and early teens. Interestingly, this rate drop disappears when youth with CD who also meet ODD criteria are not excluded from consideration.

Maughan and colleagues' (2004) analysis was consistent with similar surveys from around the world in that there was a high degree of comorbidity in both CD and ODD. Thirty-six percent of girls and 46 percent of boys with ODD met criteria for at least one other disorder that was not in the DBD family. Thirty-nine percent of girls and 46 percent of boys with CD met criteria for at least one other mental disorder that was not in the DBD family (Connor & Doerfler, 2008).

Overall, attention deficit hyperactivity disorder (ADHD) was the most highly comorbid diagnosis with both ODD and CD. This has been suggested by other studies indicating that ADHD was most highly associated with girls with CD, but these data fell just short of reaching statistical significance (e.g., p value of 0.6) (Keenan et al., 1999). Maughan and colleagues astutely raise the question of whether girls may require a greater allostatic load in order to develop CD. Also noteworthy, boys and girls with ODD and/or who met criteria for both ODD and CD were more likely to have comorbid mental disorders (e.g., ADHD, depression, anxiety) than youth who had CD alone. In all, CD, and most likely ODD, are more common in boys. Both display a high degree of comorbidity with other mental disorders, especially ADHD.

In the case of ADHD, comorbid ODD or CD can have synergistic effects on the severity of a young person's difficulties. In 2008 Connor and colleagues showed that ADHD severity rose in stair-step fashion from ADHD alone, to ADHD with comorbid ODD, and ADHD with accompanying CD (Connor & Doerfler, 2008). Burke, Rowe, and Boylan (2014) elucidated how a childhood diagnosis of ODD in boys that persists into adolescence is associated with significant reductions in social functioning during young adulthood. The boys involved in this prospective study were identified between the ages of 7 and 12 as having a diagnosis of ODD, followed yearly up to age 18, and then once more at age 24. Those with ODD symptoms that persisted through age 18 tended to have poorer quality romantic relationships and more troubled relationships with their fathers, and they were less likely to have favorable job recommendations at age 24. Youth with ODD who went on to develop CD were also shown to have a host of problems in young adulthood that included being more prone to sustaining violent injuries, reduced academic achievement, and workplace problems.

3.2.3 DBDS IN CLINICAL POPULATIONS

Given our estimates of prevalence of DBDs, we can now understand why they are the most common referring complaint for pediatric psychiatric consultation and often account for between 25% to 90% of requests in some clinics. This stands in contrast to the general population prevalence of disruptive patterns, which varies between 1.5% to 20%, again depending on definitions and methods of data collection (Connor, 2002). Notably, these behaviors, at least in their overt form, are highly skewed toward males with male-to-female ratios ranging between 3:1 and 5:1 (Cohen et al., 1993). Recent research is beginning to uncover a different pattern for girls; it is becoming evident that social aggression and more covert forms of aggressive behavior may be present for females (Celio, Karnik, & Steiner, 2006; Hawkins, Miller, & Steiner, 2003). It is quite likely that our studies of aggression in children may underreport these types of aggression, relative to the more traditional forms of physical aggression and disruptive behaviors seen in boys (Hawkins et al., 2003).

A subset of these children go on to develop maladaptive patterns of disruptive behaviors that merit clinical attention. Current estimates show that when applying DSM-IV criteria in a general population, sample roughly 1.8% of children meet criteria for ODD, while 3.2% will meet ICD-10 standards for ODD (Rowe, Maughan, Costello, & Angold, 2005). Psychiatric epidemiologists have noted that the ICD-10 definition more effectively captures children who are having clinically significant behavioral issues.

CD appears to also be present in about 2% of children at any given time, but ages of these children are markedly older than those with ODD (Rowe et al., 2005). Using the ICD standard it is apparent that a cohort of children may progress from ODD to CD. Strict DSM-IV criteria do not capture this transition well.

The finding of 2% seems to be a relatively stable percentage with a study from the British National Child Mental Health Study finding CD at a rate of 2.1% in boys and 0.8% in girls (Maughan et al., 2004). While specific DSM epidemiological studies would be beneficial, seeking and finding these studies can be challenging, as burdens to these studies include the required length of time for set up and results or outcomes. Despite this, the BELLA study out of Germany has been able to provide some data. Having surveyed 2,863 families with children ages 7 to 17, the BELLA study screened for a variety of mental health diagnoses, including suicidality and substance abuse. Prevalence data revealed that 8.6% of the children in this group and 6.6% of adolescents endorsed issues with mental health. This data gleaned from Germany reveals that mental health issues begin early and are definitely worthy of significant early intervention; less than half of the reported children and adolescents were receiving treatment (Ravens-Sieberer et al., 2008).

3.2.4 A GLIMPSE OF ONE PATHWAY INTO DBDS: THE ROLE OF MALTREATMENT

It has long been suggested that childhood trauma and family dysfunction have cumulative effects on young peoples' development. Felitti and colleagues (1998), in their groundbreaking large-scale retrospective study, set about the task of quantifying the relationship between the number and types of exposures to adverse childhood experiences with long-term physical and mental health outcomes. Not surprisingly, adults with more traumatic upbringings tended to experience greater levels of alcoholism, depression, drug abuse, and poor physical health. This study helped pave the way for similar attempts to look at the relationship between childhood experiences, mental disorders among youth, and their comorbidities (Nock, Kazdin, Hiripi, & Kessler, 2006, 2007).

In the early 2000s, the National Comorbidity Survey Replication (NCS-R) retrospectively examined mental disorders among 3,199 Americans between the ages of 18 and 44. Nearly half (i.e., 46%) of the participants in the NCS-R who had met criteria for ODD during their youth had also met criteria for a mood disorder at some point during their lifetime. Individuals with a history of ODD had a lifetime prevalence of major depressive disorder (MDD) of 39%. The lifetime prevalence of bipolar disorder among NCS-R participants with a history of ODD was 20%. Anxiety disorders were even more prevalent among the ODD group, with over 60% of them reporting that they suffered from an anxiety disorder at one time. The most prevalent anxiety disorders among the

ODD group were PTSD, social phobia, and specific phobia. Approximately one-half of the ODD group who met criteria reported a lifetime history of one or more substance use disorders. Just over one-third of the ODD group reported a history of being diagnosed with ADHD, while around two-fifths of those with ODD also reported a diagnosis of CD. One bright spot for the ODD group was the data indicating that the risk of developing new mental disorders reduced significantly, once ODD had resolved.

Individuals with a history of CD who participated in the NCS-R showed dramatically increased rates of substance use disorders, mood disorders (e.g., MDD and bipolar disorder), anxiety disorders, ADHD, obsessive-compulsive disorder, and intermittent explosive disorder. In most cases, the development of CD preceded that of subsequent mood disorders and/or substance use disorders. Alternatively, ODD, ADHD, and intermittent explosive disorder tended to develop before CD among those surveyed in the NCS-R who reported a previous diagnosis of CD. Similar to the ODD group, co-occurring mental disorders were most likely to be present in those with active symptoms of CD.

To summarize this chapter's empirical discussion, we have yet to test the impact of the changes of DBD criteria and grouping in the DSM and ICD in independent and rigorous studies. Judging by past studies examining these issues in the previous iterations, we might see a change in the prevalence and incidence numbers. Changes in prevalence and incidence can occur in response to increased diagnostic rigor by looking for more symptoms and adding frequency and severity requirements. We also are in great need of incidence studies. We need to know how many new cases of DBDs emerge per unit of time to accurately gauge the resources needed to manage them properly and to examine potential economic and historical effects.

The ICD and DSM are increasingly making the exact criteria for DBDs identical. We are supportive of this effort. What is still needed is an empirical comparison of the two systems' different way of grouping DBDs. The current grouping in the ICD makes more sense from a developmental point of view.

3.3 Implications for Clinical Practice

When a youngster presents for an evaluation due to concerns related to aggressive behaviors, the clinician must have a solid grasp of what normative developmental aggression looks like. The infant/toddler stage has been previously discussed in chapter 2. The preschool stage has been well characterized by Gerald Patterson and colleagues of the Oregon Social Learning Center. Patterson and colleagues describe how children begin to realize that they are able to act in ways that Mom and Dad are not able to control, leading to what's known as a "coercive cycle."

This realization on the child's part and the interactions that result are important because it is when the youth realizes that he or she is an individual with a certain degree of autonomy. In other words, the child realizes that she is the captain of her own ship and that she can choose to sail alongside mom and dad or break ranks. If said child grows up in an environment with overly permissive parenting and learns that she can go her own way without consequences, behavioral problems are often not far behind. By the same token, if a parent manages a child's expression of individuality by harsh or even abusive parenting, this also will lead to major problems later on. Managing children's antisocial or aggressive behavior by attacking them models all the wrong ideas. We discuss this in more detail in chapters 4 and 5 on etiology and treatment, respectively (Patterson, 1982; Patterson, Reid, & Dishion, 1992).

Before grade school, kids are primarily capable of hot aggression. However, a child exposed to overly permissive parenting practices may begin to show some concerning new behaviors in grade school. This is because, as the frontal lobes mature, so does a child's ability to control impulses, calculate, and plan. In our view, overly permissive parenting can set the stage for acts of planned cold aggression that the child sees as justifiable. The forms of cold aggression kids display during the early grade school years tend to be somewhat clumsy in their execution. That said, by the time early adolescence arrives we begin to see the emergence of gender differences in which girls often become much more covertly aggressive and boys more overtly aggressive.

We often notice a difference in how different clinicians, mental health, and medical subspecialties deal with aggression that presents in the mid- to late teen years. As has been reported in the consultation liaison literature and as we have experienced in our own practice consulting to primary care providers, there is a risk of normalizing behavioral problems such as constitute DBDs. This is completely understandable, because the primary care point of view is different from that of a mental health specialist, who may err on the side of pathologizing behaviors. It is at this difficult juncture that a mental health clinician is left to determine if the reported aggression fits into or outside of a normative pattern. In the following we describe some cases to make this decision more clear, as we continue to examine clinical practice implications.

An illustrative example is the case of an 11-year-old daughter of an immigrant mother and Asian father. Upon gathering information from the school, it was reported that the mother expressed concern that her daughter was not doing her chores or homework and was falling behind in school with poor grades. The school did not corroborate that this information was different from the behavior they had witnessed during the school days. The child was experiencing significant pressure at home from her father, who was expecting nothing less than straight As. The dilemma with this expectation was that his daughter was not a studious girl, in addition to high suspicion of undiagnosed learning problems. Her father insisted that she participate in an accelerated learning track at school, with goals of her attending a prestigious private high school and matriculating at his alma mater, Johns Hopkins University.

Upon examination, when the girl walked into the room she was extremely deferential, authority oriented, and exhibited high eye flutter rate with a moist handshake. This anxious presentation was further supported with a resting heart rate of 115 bpm and an elevated blood pressure of 135/85 (normal is 120/80). It was clear from her breathing pattern that she was extremely anxious, which persisted throughout the interview. Psychometric assessments, including the BASC-2, revealed endorsement of almost all internalizing symptoms. This is quite contrary from the externalizing symptoms parents reported seeing at home. This is an extremely common scenario, when a clinician is required to first establish and acknowledge externalizing behaviors, then look closely for the internalizing disorder that drives the externalizing symptoms. While treatment will be discussed in later chapters, for completeness we briefly touch on further formulation of this case. Her father was a "tiger father," whom the child found to be unhelpful, with a primary requirement of timely homework completion, resulting in good grades. Her mother was chaotic and disorganized, likely with her own anxiety symptoms. This set the stage for this patient's externalizing presentation for evaluation. A case of pure ODD that is not comorbid may sometimes be the result of a lack of parent training. This particular case highlights two ways in which parenting can go awry: abusive parenting and permissive parenting. Either pathway is equally strong in producing noncompliant, oppositional children. Overlapping anxiety and ODD, as previously discussed in chapter 2 and demonstrated with this case, usually presents when there is an increase in academic demand. Most externalizing symptoms are usually picked up in school-age children, while the "triple threat" of internalizing, externalizing, and ODD or CD tend to be found in older children. Oftentimes, they have been in some sort of treatment but has not been completed, for a variety of reasons. This could be likened to what we have learned from the ADHD literature, in that as ADHD children grow older, it becomes increasingly difficult to blame others for the trouble they are having, and as soon as that manifests as true it makes them anxious because they recognize that something is not "right." In some ways, this translates as a risk for them, but it can be helpful, as it is from that point they truly become patients.

In order to identify and diagnose problems with antisocial and aggressive behavior very early in the process, the clinician needs to be aware of any developmental risk factors and antecedents to actual disorders. As we discuss in more detail in chapter 4 on etiology, there are many that deserve our attention: temperament, constitution, attachment, parenting styles, academic performance, and family subculture/environment. This work usually happens in collaboration with primary care and a presence in schools. Such collaborations and consultations are so important because most of the prevention and intervention literature in DBDs shows that the earlier we intervene, the greater the chances are that we will be able to help the patient. And primary care doctors and school personnel are in an excellent position by virtue of their professional role to be the first to notice problems in this area. We address this issue in some detail in chapter 5 on treatment.

Generally, there seems to be a prejudice among parents and professionals that problems with antisocial and aggressive behavior are more prevalent in boys. We have a fair amount of information on this issue across the developmental age span. In preschool, there are very few gender differences, especially when we are dealing with infants and toddlers. This equality seems to persist into school-age children. Recently, a 10-year-old girl presented to our clinic with her parents reporting a several-year history of oppositional behavior toward adults, including teachers, friends' parents, and her own parents. She became a challenge for discipline per her parents and exhibited a number of oppositional and negative behaviors including frequent lying, stealing from her siblings and peers, and being overly aggressive with her younger and older siblings. In hearing the description of her, as presented by her parents, other than given the identifying gender information, one might have assumed her gender to be male. This girl presented for evaluation one to two years shy of potentially developing additional complicating symptoms for which she was at risk secondary to her externalizing symptoms. However, under the impact of maturation and puberty, girls initially become more internalizing, displaying elements of anxiety, sadness, and self-deprecating attitudes. In contrast, boys become more boisterous, highlighting these gender differences to a greater degree. As puberty progresses, though, there is some closure in the gender gap (Hawkins et al., 2003). Much of this is due to what has been termed "social aggression," which is more of the covert and coldly planned variety and aims at attacking other girls by rumor and spreading suspicion.

This pattern changes as we examine gender differences among delinquent populations: as we discuss in some detail in chapter 6 on forensics, there is a wide gap between girl and boy offenders. This may be due to many factors, among them the relative ease with which delinquent girls are managed in less restrictive settings and differential adjudication practices driven by court prejudices. For example, judges tend to give more girls the benefit of the doubt; or institutional delinquent care has different availability dependent on gender. Most established institutions are for male delinquents (Karnik et al., 2009).

The cases presented specifically address those children presenting from a community clinic sample. One will find a much different type of DBD presentation in the juvenile justice setting. While this will be addressed in the forensic chapter to come, let us at least introduce the concept of high eco-logical validity. We revisit our initial definition of epidemiology as defined by the Stedman dictionary: Epidemiology is "the investigation and application of trends, distribution and causation pertinent to particular groups or popu-lations with regards to health care or specific events" (Stedman, 2006). This maps on to the groups we have discussed among the general population as well as the juvenile justice population.

High ecological validity refers to the fact that DBDs are indeed found in high numbers in populations which should have high frequencies of DBDs, that is, delinquents, youth who have committed many and sometimes very severe antisocial and aggressive acts. Finding many DBDs in such lends considerable validity to the very concepts underlying DBDs. Given our uncertainty as to the validity of DBDs other than interrater agreement induced by standardizing cri-teria for DBDs, such a finding gives us some assurance that we are on the right track as we introduce the world of medicine and developmental psychiatry into the world of law and justice. We discuss this point in more detail in chapter 6 on forensics. To illustrate, though, how the presentation of DBDs can be quite different in juvenile justice settings—much more confusing and complex—we discuss an illustrative case.

A 12-year-old Caucasian boy is raised by his single alcoholic mother along-side his gang-involved older brother in a mobile home community, complicated by spotty school attendance. He has poor grades, an academic history pointing to long-standing learning challenges, and severe ADHD. He has had two prior offenses at school when he climbed onto the roof after school hours, and the other when he was caught tagging. In efforts to emulate his older brother (recently taken into custody for car theft), he begins to befriend a suspicious group at school. One of his friends within the group brings a knife to school, which quickly becomes an opportunity to gain attention from peers, in particular a group of girls they are interested in. This boy takes things a step further as he impulsively grabs one of the girls, wrapping his arm around her neck from behind and holding the knife to her neck, telling her he is going to cut her throat. Startled and afraid, the girl quickly retreats from his grasp, yells at him to get lost, which enrages the young perpetrator. He had been overheard bragging to his friends about how tough and scary he is. He clearly fulfills criteria of CD and other diagnoses, but the crucial question is why was he enraged in reaction to the girl's rejecting him? Why was he not contrite and apologetic? Does he lack an understanding of the rules of conviviality? How did this situation escalate so quickly for him? How could one help explain his deeds to a court, to a worried principal, and, most important, to the victim?

After many sessions in treatment the answers to these questions began to emerge. The notion of being rejected by a woman was not unfamiliar to him.

As the history continues to unfold we uncover an even more traumatic history of being rejected and threatened by his alcoholic mother endlessly during critical times of development within his life. Naturally, any rejection from another female quickly takes him back to his own trauma, activating a variety of physiological and psychological triggers for him.

This boy is an example of a very complicated case involving the internalizing symptoms pointing to PTSD, externalizing problems, learning problems, and more. The clinician should not expect to obtain all this information after a single visit. These are the types of cases that require in-depth evaluation over time. Through confirmation of his traumatic antecedents, which in part explain his extreme reactions to a relatively innocuous social situation, a therapeutic alliance can be established. After many sessions the boy reveals a candid history of his older sister, who used to invite her friends over. They would tease him and badger him with borderline sexually abusive antics. Courting and intimacy became instruments of domination and threat, not avenues of security and pleasure. The clinician in the juvenile justice setting has to expect such complicated layers of internalizing and externalizing disorders, which come to light only after much work and re-education. Fortunately we have at our disposal an incremental data base that adequately prepares us for many of the eventualities as we practice in juvenile justice settings.

In concluding this chapter there are a few take-away points that many readers may find useful for their clinical practice. It is important for clinicians to remain alert as youth with DBDs are particularly prone to receiving inaccurate diagnoses that can lead to delays in proper treatment. We contend that our field's continued attempts at diagnostic clarity and decisiveness via the DSM-5 and ICD-10, while helpful in some ways, may not be ideal. Only time and experience will tell how well our classification schemes will evolve to become more useful for the diagnosis and treatment of DBDs. We are in great need of more carefully documented number of prevalence, incidence, and ecological validity from more ideally structured studies. These include large samples from the general population, school populations, clinical populations, and juvenile justice populations. The instrumentation used should be increasingly specific, going from broad-based, sensitive screens, to probing follow-up studies with specific interview and clinical measures in high- and low-risk subsamples. These studies then should be tied to extensive prospective follow-up to document validity of diagnoses, cohesion of grouping, switches between diagnostic categories, breeding true of categories, and differentiation or lack thereof of categories. This is an ambitious program not to be competed quickly and easily. The ultimate goal though, to ameliorate the world of justice through the presence of medicine is very much worth it.

References

American Psychiatric Association. (2000). *Diagnostic and statistical manual of mental disorders*, 4th ed., text rev. Washington, DC: Author.

Belsky, J., Vandell, D. L., Burchinal, M., Clarke-Stewart, K. A., McCartney, K., & Owen, M. T. (2007). Are there long-term effects of early child care? *Child Development, 78*(2), 681–701.

Burke, J. D., Rowe, R., & Boylan, K. (2014). Functional outcomes of child and adolescent oppositional defiant disorder symptoms in young adult men. *Journal of Child Psychology and Psychiatry, 55*(3), 264–272.

Celio, M., Karnik, N. S., & Steiner, H. (2006). Early maturation as a risk factor for aggression and delinquency in adolescent girls: A review. *International Journal of Clinical Practice, 60*(10), 1254–1262.

Cohen, P., Cohen, J., Kasen, S., Velez, C. N., Hartmark, C., Johnson, J., . . . Streuning, E. L. (1993). An epidemiological study of disorders in late childhood and adolescence—I. Age- and gender-specific prevalence. *Journal of Child Psychology and Psychiatry, 34*(6), 851–867.

Connor, D. F. (2002). *Aggression and antisocial behavior in children and adolescents: Research and treatment*. New York: Guilford Press.

Connor, D. F., & Doerfler, L. A. (2008). ADHD with comorbid oppositional defiant disorder or conduct disorder: Discrete or nondistinct disruptive behavior disorders? *Journal of Attention Disorders, 12*(2), 126–134. doi:10.1177/1087054707308486

Felitti, V. J., Anda, R. F., Nordenberg, D., Williamson, D. F., Spitz, A. M., Edwards, V., . . . Marks, J. S. (1998). Relationship of childhood abuse and household dysfunction to many of the leading causes of death in adults: The Adverse Childhood Experiences (ACE) Study. *American Journal of Preventive Medicine, 14*(4), 245–258.

Hawkins, S. R., Miller, S. P., & Steiner, H. (2003). Aggression, psychopathology, and delinquency: Influences of gender and maturation—where did all the good girls go? In C. Hayward (Ed.), *Gender differences at puberty* (pp. 93–112). Cambridge, UK: Cambridge University Press.

Karnik, N. S., Popma, A., Blair, J., Khanzode, L., P. Miller, S., & Steiner, H. (2008). Personality correlates of physiological response to stress among incarcerated juveniles. *Zeitschrift für Kinder- und Jugendpsychiatrie und Psychotherapie, 36*(3), 185–190.

Karnik, N. S., Soller, M., Redlich, A., Silverman, M., Kraemer, H. C., Haapanen, R., & Steiner, H. (2009). Prevalence of and gender differences in psychiatric disorders among juvenile delinquents incarcerated for nine months. *Psychiatric Services, 60*(6), 838–841.

Maughan, B., Rowe, R., Messer, J., Goodman, R., & Meltzer, H. (2004). Conduct disorder and oppositional defiant disorder in a national sample: Developmental epidemiology. *Journal of Child Psychology and Psychiatry, 45*(3), 609–621.

NICHD Early Child Care Research Network, & Arsenio, W. F. (2004). Trajectories of physical aggression from toddlerhood to middle childhood: Predictors, correlates, and outcomes. *Monographs of the Society for Research in Child Development, 69*(4), i–143.

Nock, M. K., Kazdin, A. E., Hiripi, E., & Kessler, R. C. (2006). Prevalence, subtypes, and correlates of DSM-IV conduct disorder in the National Comorbidity Survey Replication. *Psychologial Medicine, 36*(5), 699–710. doi:10.1017/s0033291706007082

Nock, M. K., Kazdin, A. E., Hiripi, E., & Kessler, R. C. (2007). Lifetime prevalence, correlates, and persistence of oppositional defiant disorder: Results from the National Comorbidity Survey Replication. *Journal of Child Psychology and Psychiatry, 48*(7), 703–713.

Patterson, G. (1982). Coercive family process. Eugene: Castalia. Patterson, GR (2002). The early development of coercive family processes. *Antisocial behavior in children and adolescents: A developmental analysis and model for intervention*, 2544.

Patterson, G. R., Reid, J. B., & Dishion, T. J. (1992). *Antisocial boys: A social interactional approach*. Eugene, OR: Castalia.

Ravens-Sieberer, U., Wille, N., Erhart, M., Bettge, S., Wittchen, H.-U., Rothenberger, A., . . . Döpfner, M. (2008). Prevalence of mental health problems among children and adolescents in Germany: Results of the BELLA study within the National Health Interview and Examination Survey. *European Child & Adolescent Psychiatry*, 17(1), 22–33. doi:10.1007/s00787-008-1003-2

Rowe, R., Maughan, B., Costello, E. J., & Angold, A. (2005). Defining oppositional defiant disorder. *Journal of Child Psychology and Psychiatry*, 46(12), 1309–1316.

Stedman, T. L. (2006). *Stedman's medical dictionary*. Baltimore: Lippincott Williams & Wilkins.

Steiner, H. (2011). *Handbook of developmental psychiatry*. London: World Scientific.

Steiner, H., & Hall, R. E. (2015). *Treating adolescents*. Hoboken, NJ: John Wiley.

Steiner, H., Silverman, M., Karnik, N. S., Huemer, J., Plattner, B., Clark, C. E., . . . Haapanen, R. (2011). Psychopathology, trauma and delinquency: Subtypes of aggression and their relevance for understanding young offenders. *Child and Adolescent Psychiatry and Mental Health*, 5(1), 21.

Suggested Readings and Resources

Eaton, W. W., & Kessler, L. G. (2012). *Epidemiologic field methods in psychiatry: The NIMH Epidemiologic Catchment Area Program*. New York: Academic Press.

Excellence, N. I. f. C. (2013). *Antisocial behaviour and conduct disorders in children and young people: Recognition, intervention and management*. NICE Clinical Guideline 158. Washington, DC: National Institute for Health and Care Excellence.

Fatemi, S. H. (2013). Textbook of psychiatric epidemiology. *Journal of Clinical Psychiatry*, 74(1), 118–118.

Haapanen, R., & Steiner, H. (2003). *Identifying mental health treatment needs among serious institutionalized delinquents using paper-and-pencil screening instruments, final report*. Washington, DC: US Department of Justice, Office of Justice Program, National Institute of Justice.

Keenan, K., Loeber, R., & Green, S. (1999). Conduct disorder in girls: A review of the literature. *Clinical Child and Family Psychology Review*, 2(1), 3–19.

Offord, D. R., Boyle, M. H., & Racine, Y. (1989). Ontario child health study: Correlates of disorder. *Journal of the American Academy of Child & Adolescent Psychiatry*, 28(6), 856–860.

Robins, L. N., & Price, R. K. (1991). Adult disorders predicted by childhood conduct problems: Results from the NIMH Epidemiologic Catchment Area project. *Psychiatry*, 54(2), 116–132.

Schachar, R., Rutter, M., & Smith, A. (1981). The characteristics of situationally and pervasively hyperactive children: Implications for syndrome definition. *Journal of Child Psychology and Psychiatry*, 22(4), 375–392.

Steiner, H. (1997). Practice parameters for the assessment and treatment of children and adolescents with conduct disorder. *Journal of the American Academy of Child & Adolescent Psychiatry*, 36(10), 122S–139S.

Steiner, H., & Remsing, L. (2007). Practice parameter for the assessment and treatment of children and adolescents with oppositional defiant disorder. *Journal of the American Academy of Child & Adolescent Psychiatry*, 46(1), 126–141.

Swanson, J. W., Holzer, C. E. III, Ganju, V. K., & Jono, R. T. (1990). Violence and psychiatric disorder in the community: Evidence from the Epidemiologic Catchment Area surveys. *Psychiatric Services*, 41(7), 761–770.

4

Etiology of Disruptive
Behavior Disorders

4.1 Definitions

Etiology : "the science and study of the causes of disease and their mode of operation" (Stedman, 2006).

The goal in medicine is to arrive at a complete knowledge of the causes that drive diseases in order to disrupt or correct them. The knowledge of these mechanisms allows the physician to match interventions onto what is needed to restore health and give us the highest chance of good treatment outcomes.

Our current knowledge regarding the etiology of disruptive behavior disorders (DBDs) is neither complete nor definitive. This problem is driven by the complexity of the problems involved; the heterogeneity of each of the main diagnoses in this grouping; and the fact that children, adolescents, and adults are moving targets—that is, their domains of functioning that are impacted by disease processes are not static. They change as a function of maturation, development, and normal aging. Domains of functioning go from being undifferentiated to differentiated. Differentiated states are usually more static and less dynamic in their essence, which makes it easier for researchers and clinicians to study them and arrive at valid conclusions regarding their nature and the treatment needed to correct them.

Pathogenesis: "the pathologic, physiologic, or biochemical mechanism resulting in the development of disease or morbid process" (Stedman, 2006).

As is, this definition of etiology focuses on physiological or biological mechanisms and causes of disease, but it does not exclude other factors that, as we will see, are relevant in the study of DBDs, such as social and psychological processes gone awry.

In previous publications, we have repeatedly suggested in our discussions of DBDs the array of relevant factors to be considered in the study, the research, and the clinical practice of DBDs. Figure 4.1 provides a schema that emphasizes

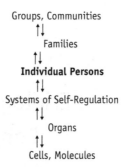

Figure 4.1 Levels of organization relevant to research and clinical practice in DBDs.

the relevant factors. DBDs viewed from a developmental psychiatry perspective are caused by entities that match this wide range of factors. Cells and molecules and their constituents should be informative, as we improve our understanding of how biological risks such as differing levels of neurotransmitters and related biochemical compounds active in neurotransmission can lead to higher levels of risk taking and future aggression. Most of our current studies in psychopharmacology rely on this information. Organs, such as the amygdala and the medial orbitofrontal lobes, are implicated in problems with empathy and callous–unemotional traits. Systems of self-regulation, such as the threat detection system or the attachment system, have been shown to influence effortful self-control and planned antisocial acts. On the level of individual characteristics and personality, there are increasingly strong data that certain character traits—callous–unemotional, for instance—are associated with DBDs and psychopathy. At the level of family, we know that parenting strongly influences the emergence of DBDs, as Gerald Patterson's work has shown, and at the levels of groups and communities, we know that lack of structure and criminogenic influences heavily influence youths to take deviant pathways toward DBDs, especially during adolescence. As we will see in chapter 5, all of these mechanisms have been implicated in preclinical and clinical studies. They offer promising windows into cause, diagnosis, intervention, and prevention.

The dilemma for the practitioner is how to assign primacy to the entire array of processes we list in Figure 4.1 in order to deliver appropriately matched and effective treatments. The descriptive systems we discussed in chapter 2 at some length fail to help in this regard. They treat processes as divergent as "forced sexual acts on another" and "lying for secondary gain" as equivalent criteria for the diagnosis of conduct disorder. Upon further reflection, we can easily see that the former probably has a much closer relationship to biology (Tanner status, sexual arousal, pairing of arousal with stressful arousal, etc.). By contrast, lying for secondary gain (a more planned, strategic, premeditated, instrumental behavior) seems intuitively more related to processes such as low levels of self-assurance and self-esteem (psychological) or mistrust of others to provide what one desires or the world being unfairly discriminating because of certain ethnic or other social hierarchy motives (social). Giving someone medications for non-normative sexual behavior and needs would presumably do very little for his or her need to lie for personal gain. Lying is generally regarded as an instrumental (planned) from of antisocial behavior, carefully crafted and controlled, while sexual assault most often is emotionally induced and facilitated by disinhibited states, such as inebriation. We have to go beneath the surface in order to match intervention to symptoms(s) and diagnoses to be effective. These distinctions are not just an intellectual exercise for the clinician.

Cause: "the person or thing that gives rise to an action, phenomenon or condition" (Merriam-Webster, 2006).

Again, this definition does not restrict the meaning of the term to biology. Psychiatry, as the discipline in medicine that is in the most prominent position of straddling the social, psychological, and biological sciences, needs to avoid any premature orthodoxy leading to a restrictive reductionism. All of medicine, as an applied discipline dealing with individuals, is in this difficult and challenging position. This is clear as we approach such problems as pain, compliance with treatment, and prevention of disease, which all call on the physician to draw on the entire range of biopsychosocial interventions. Likewise, this is also true in the study and treatment of DBDs. The question is, once again, how to create a theory that supports the serious consideration necessary for the full range of biopsychosocial dimensions of disease and disorder, without falling prey to a pernicious reductionism that does not serve the patient well. On the other hand, we also need to remind ourselves that reductionism is an excellent tool for research. Based on Occam's razor, it is the basis for many important empirical and clinical findings. By contrast, clinicians are usually not well served by this attitude. They do not deal with cells and neurons; they deal with patients, whole persons, individuals. It is tempting to fall into the trap of reductionism to gain respect of some of our colleagues and patients. But to think in a reductionist way does not serve us well in the consulting room, as the barren research of "biological markers" where psychopathology is reduced to simple biological mechanisms demonstrates. Just remember the flurry of excitement when the dexamethasone suppression test was considered the diagnostic tool for depression; when bipolar disorder was reduced to a relatively simple genetic defect; when schizophrenia was a malfunction of the dopamine neurotransmitter system. DBDs in some ways are even more complex disorders than these. It is highly doubtful that the complex psychopathology captured in the DBD grouping will ever be successfully reduced to a handful of biological variables.

Developmental psychopathology: the study of the processes leading to mental disorders. There is a strong emphasis on studying normal and abnormal development simultaneously, as they both inform each other. Developmental psychiatry is an extension of this theory into psychiatric practice (Steiner & Hall, 2015). Developmental psychopathology offers several helpful tools to approach the study, diagnosis, and treatment of DBDs. These tools are of special interest to the developmental psychiatrist. First, developmental change is influenced by many variables. The logical research and clinical designs should therefore be multivariate. Second, development does not occur in a vacuum but in what Bronfenbrenner (1986) has labeled "nested contexts." These are contexts that reach from family to community to society, all of which can have a positive or negative impact on a child. Thus development arises from a dynamic interplay of physiological, genetic, social, cognitive, emotional, and cultural influences across time.

Conduct disorder is often considered a great example of an disorder that is best explained by the developmental psychopathology approach (Leve & Cicchetti, 2016; Steiner, 2004, 2011; Steiner & Hall, 2015). Conduct disorder (and most likely other diagnoses in the DBD cluster) starts out with many behaviors that are quite common and progressively worsen as the child gets older, to the point where the behavior deteriorates and becomes pathological, ultimately progressing into syndromal disorder, which can be diagnosed (Gerald Patterson, personal communication). Such a pattern of pathogenesis fits developmental psychopathology well, because one of its cardinal tenets is that psychopathology can be best understood as normal development gone awry, like Figure 4.2 indicates. Every human comes into this world with a given set of factors—deficits and capacities—which after birth get shaped by the environments he or she grows up in. DBDs most likely follow this pattern and can best be understood as a sequence of genetic loading, which then is shaped by gene–environment interactions in the process of growing up. As we discuss in some detail later and as we have discussed in the chapter on epidemiology, we have prospective data from New Zealand that support this idea. So, for instance, a child may be born with either a high or low set range of arousal.

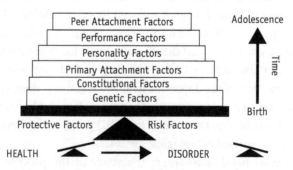

Figure 4.2 The risk/resilience factor model of DBDs.

Depending on whether he or she is raised in a high or low criminogenic environment, this genetically set range will put him or her at a higher or lower risk of a DBD outcome. This is one of the main tenets in developmental psychiatry: genetic factors do not just simply drive us into psychopathology. They pose certain risks for our development but are not determining outcomes a priori. Gene–environment interactions abound.

In this schema, we add another feature that will be helpful for understanding the complex situation we find ourselves in when we study, research, diagnose, and treat DBDs. Figure 4.2 shows our vulnerability/resilience model for the development of DBDs. The model shows crucial factors (not an exhaustive list) relevant to the etiology of DBDs and their ascendance in importance as development proceeds. Mental health is exemplified by a balance beam, sitting on a narrow fulcrum. Going forward from birth, humans acquire increasing capacities and abilities in various domains, which potentially confer risk for and offer protection from the development of DBDs. As these factors become evident and functional, they keep the balance between resilience and psychopathology, provided they are present in normative amounts and function well. In the course of development, any hypotrophy or dysfunction of any of these factors can tilt the balance beam in the direction of disorder. To reestablish mental health, or perhaps even resilience, the clinician needs to target the specific sets of factors in an effective way. The list of factors ranges from genetic to other constitutional factors, attachment, personality, academic and vocational performance, and peer attachment. The list is not meant to be complete, simply illustrative.

The vulnerability/resilience model also suggests an age-relative relevance of the factors: the younger the child, the more genetic and constitutional, temperamental factors are important. Peer factors barely exist. In adolescence, though, the model suggests that early biological factors recede in importance, while we see the full impact of performance potential, positive response to demands from others, and forming and retention of a positive peer group. This schema also suggests that we cannot expect dramatic changes in response to interventions in a case where there has been a great deal of increasing risk of moving the bar into the disorder direction. As an example, the idea that simple 12-week group intervention in adolescence—often used in diversion programs—would offset years of cumulative risk in constitution, attachment, personality, and academic performance is simply unrealistic. Similarly, expecting that there will be a very potent effect of medications increasing self-regulation and control, bringing about extensive changes in the delinquent peer group affiliation of an individual growing up in an abusive family, is unrealistic. Compare also the Joachim Puig-Antich findings in the 1980s regarding similar expected effects of treating juvenile depression with tricyclics. The medications helped with sleep, appetite, concentration, and mood but failed to alter the highly avoidant peer behavior often associated with depression. Depressed juveniles felt better on a basic level of functioning, but this did not automatically translate into better peer relationships. Psychotherapy was needed to address this problem in addition to medication. We expect a very similar outcome in DBDs.

4.2 Review of the Recent Relevant Literature

As of now, it is difficult to assign definitive causes to the pathogenesis of DBDs and their subtypes due to the heterogenous nature of our DBD diagnostic categories whose discriminant and predictive validity are unknown. As our discussion of the current literature will show, we have good candidates—many mental health subdomains of biological, psychological, and social factors that ultimately should provide an answer for us, provided we carry out the necessary studies. But for now, we are uncertain as to which level of causal factors we should concentrate on, which give us the best opportunity to intervene effectively, which hold the greatest promise for which diagnosis in this grouping, and which will lead us to the best way to subtype the large and heterogenous categories of almost all the DBDs, helping us define the diagnoses more crisply and decisively. This state of affairs leads us to the decision to divide the causal factors into the three domains of the biopsychosocial model. We retain that tripartite division in Chapter 5 in order to show how to match the most relevant interventions onto what we know to be causal factors in DBDs. The eclecticism in our treatment of these disorders is simply a reflection of our state of ignorance (or knowledge, if one prefers).

As has been our mantra thus far, it is our opinion that description in the *Diagnostic and Statistical Manual of Mental Disorders* (DSM) of disruptive behavior disorders and antisocial personality disorder represents a variety of behaviors with a multitude of underlying causes. As we have seen in chapters 2 and 3, youth with conduct disorders are a very heterogeneous group comprised of people with markedly varying clinical symptoms and signs and other characteristics. For instance, many youth with conduct disorder become anxious with a heightened fight-or-flight response, which in a context of maltreatment and perceived threat can result in violent behavior. Still other youth show dampened biological reactivity and less anxiety in response to stressful situations. The latter youth often have trouble empathizing with others and lack feelings of guilt following aggressive or antisocial acts. In fact, these callous–unemotional traits have also been reliably observed in youth with oppositional defiant disorder who fail to meet DSM-5 criteria for conduct disorder, yet there is no specifier in the DSM-5 identifying oppositional defiant disordered youth with callous–unemotional traits (Blair, Leibenluft, & Pine, 2014; Hawes &

Dadds, 2005; Hawes, Price, & Dadds, 2014). It is not clear from the DSM or the International Classification of Diseases (ICD) why this lack of consistency presents across the DBD diagnoses.

As best as we can glean from the existing data and newer data to be discussed, DBDs usually owe their existence to a complex series of interactions of multiple single factors and systems of adaptation that have different neurobiological, psychological, and social bases. The complexity found is also in part due to the fact that all of these systems are dynamic throughout life, changing in phenotypical manifestations across different developmental phases. Thus we need to be prepared for the absence of single-factor causality, more probable multicausality, and final common pathways fed by a varying mixture of necessary and sufficient factors. DBDs are quite distinct from diseases like strep throat (even that is a diagnosis that cannot simply be reduced to a single cause, because there is a balance between the immune system and the exposure to a noxious agent).

4.2.1 BIOLOGICAL FACTORS

The studies regarding the effects of neurobiological factors on the risk of developing DBDs' aggression and disruptive behaviors remain difficult to understand and to bring to the clinical arena. Several years ago it was shown that youth with conduct disorder have suggested deficits in several neurotransmitter systems, including serotonin (Lee & Coccaro, 2001; Swann, 2003), noradrenaline, and dopamine (Pliszka, Rogeness, Renner, Sherman, & Broussard, 1988). Our group has generated some evidence in an open trial that perhaps GABA is another neurotransmitter worthy of some attention, at least in the context of clinical risk for bipolar disorder and posttraumatic stress disorder (PTSD). Theoretically that makes sense, given that, in this open trial, levels of GABA correlated with aspects of hot aggression (Saxena, Howe, Simeonova, Steiner, & Chang, 2006). These have remained isolated studies and need further replication.

Despite the need for replication, these neurotransmitter studies have spawned an interest in looking at genetic contributions to our understanding of the neurotransmitters' role in DBDs. One question to be answered is: What are the association to several genetic vulnerabilities linked to these neurochemical systems, including the monoamine oxidase A (MAO-A) and serotonin transporter genes (5-HTT) through different pathways (Popma & Raine, 2006)? As a confirming side note, Caspi and colleagues (2003) have shown that depression tied to early life stress can be moderated by polymorphisms at the 5-HTT site. These findings have been consolidated by studies showing similar effects on the development of depression in children who have histories of maltreatment (Kaufman et al., 2006). Both of these studies and others to be discussed have supported the working model that gene–environment interactions are mutually effective and potentially have significant impacts on psychiatric illness, as developmental psychopathology would suggest (Caspi & Moffitt, 2006). We have discussed this in some detail in the preceding definitions section. These studies have implications for the selection of psychopharmacological interventions treating DBDs to be discussed in chapter 5.

Meyer-Lindenberg and colleagues (2006) looked at the effect of allelic variation in the X-linked MAO-A gene. Using a large sample of healthy adults, they observed how a low expression variant of MAO-A that is associated with aggression predicted smaller limbic structures, amygdalas that were hyperresponsive to stressful situations, and reduced activity in regions of the prefrontal cortex responsible for helping to control impulsive behaviors. The low expression version of MAO-A was also linked with reduced activation of the cingulate region of the brain during tasks involving cognitive inhibition. This study showed significant differences in neuroanatomic structures and the functional capacities related to impulsive aggression among men based on variations in the MAO-A gene (Meyer-Lindenberg et al., 2006).

In a true landmark study, Caspi and colleagues (2003) followed a birth cohort of over 1,000 youth, 52% of which were male, from childhood through young adulthood. The question to be answered was whether one could predict from genetic data who would develop antisocial behavior, having suffered abuse. The main finding was that a highly expressed version of the MAO-A gene served as a protective factor against problems related to antisocial behavior in boys who were the victims of abuse. This study provided some of the earliest evidence of how gene expression can influence resilience to trauma. A limitation of this study is that it makes no distinctions between the subtypes of aggression involved in these antisocial behaviors, nor was there an attempt to link these findings to DBDs and their subtypes. Thus we can only say that genetic vulnerability and injurious social environments lead to antisocial outcomes of differing degrees of severity. It also remains unclear what the exact relationship of these findings at the genetic level have for the various diagnostic categories grouped in the DBDs (Caspi et al., 2003).

Following the important paper by John Bowlby (1946), who was the first to suggest specifically that attachment and its disturbance could have a causal role to play in the pathogenesis of maladaptive antisocial behavior and aggression, Beitchman and colleagues (2012) hypothesized that oxytocin, a hormone associated with the formation of loving and trusting relationships, may play a role in the development of callous–unemotional traits in youth with a history of aggressive behavior. They discovered that a certain version of the oxytocin receptor (OXTR) gene was associated with youth who were particularly prone to high levels of aggression, backing up Bowlby's original findings in his clinical case series from 1944 (Beitchman et al., 2012; Bowlby, 1946).

Recent findings from a British study suggest that epigenetic factors resulting in the reduced expression of the OXTR gene is associated with reductions in circulating oxytocin levels in a subset of boys with conduct disorder and oppositional defiant disorder. In this study, the boys with conduct problems and accompanying callous–unemotional traits tended to have higher DNA methylation along particular sites in the promoter region of the OXTR gene. DNA methylation is a process that can effectively halt the expression of a particular gene. The factors that influence DNA methylation are wide ranging and include an individual's age, accompanying diseases, and even environmental factors. The process of environmental factors that do not change our genetic code yet can have major impacts on gene expression is called epigenetics. This study is exciting because it begs questions about the possible environmental factors that lead to the epigenetic changes seen in youth with callous–unemotional traits. Such an understanding would be a major step toward uncovering the genesis of callous–unemotional traits in youth and ultimately, psychopathy (Dadds, Moul, Cauchi, Dobson-Stone, Hawes, Brennan, & Ebstein, 2014).

In a related study, Dadds and colleagues (Dadds, Moul, Cauchi, Dobson-Stone, Hawes, Brennan, & Urwin, et al., 2014) also showed how variations in the promoter region of the OXTR gene were highly associated with children who exhibit disruptive behavior disorders and callous–unemotional traits. These findings are consistent with theoretical models for the development of psychopathy that link the impact oxytocin has on the cognitive and emotional differences typically seen in psychopathic individuals. (This study set also gives rise to the notion that the relationship of oxytocin to DBDs is complicated and clarified by looking simultaneously at the callous–unemotional trait.

In sum, since the earlier studies on neurotransmitter deficits in DBDs, we are moving closer to findings at the genetic/molecular level that ultimately should have implications for the biological risk factors for individuals with maladaptive antisocial and aggressive behavior. As interesting as these findings are, they have no firm diagnostic or therapeutic implications, but they deserve close follow-up in the next four to five years. A growing body of literature supports the notion that pre- and perinatal exposures can play a major role in influencing the developmental trajectories of youth due to their impact on brain regions integral to the neurocircuitry of violence and aggression (LaPrairie, Schechter, Robinson, & Brennan, 2011). These studies, if properly replicated, may also have future implications for primary care and prevention in the future. To put it simply, a mosaic of genetic vulnerabilities, perinatal insults, and environmental hardships can, in essence, result in a "perfect storm" for the development of aggressive and antisocial behavior in youth. While it is important to be aware of perinatal risk factors, we are not sure at this point which factors or combination of factors are the most relevant. In any case, from a pragmatic point of view, we cannot always prevent perinatal insults from occurring. For this reason it is important that our field continue developing strategies to address the postnatal factors that can majorly impact children's development (e.g., increasing parental access to mental health services and parenting training, programs buttressing the development of at-risk children's social skills). Fortunately, as we will discuss, there are a significant number of findings in the psychological and social domains to further guide us with regard to the diagnosis and treatment of DBDs.

4.2.2 PSYCHOLOGICAL FACTORS

In 2011, as referenced in the *Handbook of Developmental Psychiatry* (Steiner, 2011), we noticed that a wide range of psychological correlates exist for the development of aggression and disruptive behaviors such as childhood temperament (early constitutional factors), problems with learning, neuropsychological lateralization and localization (systems of systems underpinning functioning in the domains of academic and vocational achievements), and some personality traits (especially personality traits related to self-regulation and inhibition, responsibility, consideration of others, guilt and remorse, functioning under pressure while keeping negative emotions in check; Steiner, 2011).

Since then, studies have added to these findings and further expanded our understanding. Breslau, Lucia, and Alvarado (2006) recently found an association between intelligence and being able to have resiliency in the face of traumatic events, which are so common in the lives of patients with DBDs. They found that children at age six who had intelligence quotients greater than 115 were much less likely to be at lower risk from both assaultive and nonassaultive violence. These youth also had a decreased risk for the development of PTSD (Breslau, Lucia, & Alvarado, 2006). These findings are especially relevant when we consider the high rates of PTSD and dissociative symptoms in this population (Steiner, Carrion, Plattner, & Koopman, 2003; Steiner, Garcia, & Matthews, 1997).

Learning disabilities (LDs) have been well documented in the delinquent population (Grigorenko, 2006). A national survey of juvenile corrections systems has suggested that as many as 38% of the juveniles incarcerated (a population that probably has very high rates of DBDs, as we have found and discuss in detail in chapter 6) had a specific LD (Quinn, Rutherford, Leone, Osher, & Poirier, 2005). This is compared to estimates that within the nonincarcerated population, the rate of specific LDs is somewhere between 5% and 10% (Sundheim & Voeller, 2004).

A good portion of the literature examines the link between LDs and psychiatric disorders. Sundheim and Voeller (2004) report that children with language disorders are four times more likely to have externalizing disorders than children without language disorders. It is estimated that between 15% and 20% of children and adolescents with LDs will also have attention deficit hyperactivity disorder (ADHD; Halperin & McKay, 1998). This is relevant because it is increasingly recognized that there is a link between externalizing disorders and LDs, particularly deficits in verbal abilities. Studies have suggested that among children or adolescents diagnosed as having conduct disorder, or young adults diagnosed as having a personality disorder, approximately one-third have an undiagnosed or poorly treated LD (Kavale & Forness, 2000). In a study by Baker and Cantwell (1987) involving 600 children with language disabilities, 50% received a DSM diagnosis, including conduct disorder, ADHD, oppositional defiant disorder, affective disorder, or adjustment disorder. The theory that there is a possible causal connection between LDs and delinquency was proposed by Poremba in 1975.

The causal chain implies that LDs causes effects, which cause other effects, which in turn lead to delinquency (Waldie & Spreen, 1993). Brier (2001) concludes that there is likely a multifactorial explanation: that a LD is a risk factor for delinquent behavior but that other factors come into play as well. He states that individuals with LDs are more likely than non-LD individuals to display several of the language, social perception, and social relationship difficulties that have been found to contribute to the development of antisocial behavior. Important factors include early conduct problems, ADHD, low IQ, parent criminality, alcoholism, parental deficiency, and a lack of motivation to achieve (Brier, 2001).

Studies from our group show that the two subtypes of aggression—proactive/instrumental/planned (PIP) and reactive/affective/defensive/impulsive (RADI)—occur in the context of markedly different personality profiles. We have found that adolescents with a preponderance of RADI type of aggression often have high levels of anxiety and mood symptoms. In contrast, youths with high levels of PIP seem to show a pattern of underarousal and an inability to process emotions well. These youth have difficulty in understand the communication of emotion through facial characteristics and often seek aggression as a means of finding self-activation. Youth with aggressive patterns in our studies seem to have difficulty disaggregating the emotional experiences of sadness, anger, and fear especially when faced with stressful experiences (Plattner et al., 2007). This conflation experience of emotions seems to be especially dependent on prior trauma and that some trauma experiences especially in their severity and number are more potent than others.

Further understanding of the ways through which children come to act in antisocial and disruptive ways are sure to emerge in coming years from the fields of neuroscience and social cognitive science, as we study the impact of social/environmental factors on developing brains. For example, research by Bill

Greenough's group at Illinois has shown the plasticity of neuronal pathways and has begun to show the powerful effects that result from social and environmental stimuli (Grossman et al., 2003).

We are beginning to see studies of DBDs that approach the problem at the level of organ and systems dysfunction. These studies often present contradicting findings, showing how complicated it is to perform research in this area, basing recruitment on the DBD labels with methods that have a high error rate in relatively small samples. Cohn and colleagues (2015) utilized functional magnetic resonance imaging (fMRI) to observe how the process of fear extinction (i.e., the reduction in a conditioned fear response after nonreinforced exposure to a stimulus conditions to provoke a fearful response), while associated with hyperreactivity of the fear neurocircuitry when compared with healthy controls, did not differ significantly among youth with persistent disruptive behavior disorders versus those whose conduct problems resolved over time. They also found that the behavioral aspects of psychopathy (e.g., impulsiveness, irresponsibility, etc.) were particularly associated with hyperreactive responses in fear neurocircuitry (Cohn et al., 2015). Once again, operating at the level of DBD diagnoses did not show important differences, while looking at subtype characteristics such as impulsivity, which is contained in the RADI construct as well, showed a link to brain structures that are postulated to have a strong connection to emotionally charged aggression. In general, imaging studies like this are vulnerable to error due to relatively low numbers of subjects (e.g., this study involved 25 youth) and because the protocols used to record data tend to vary between studies from different research groups that are using different imaging apparatus. These are just some reasons why the replication of findings in neuroimaging studies involving mental disorders are not easily achieved.

In sum, there are several studies which—more or less successfully—are trying to link organ level dysfunctions to behavioral traits important in the diagnosis of DBDs. These findings suggest the potential utility of locating genetic and neurophysiologic variables to help identify subgroupings of youth with conduct problems. While the body of data is limited, these studies, and others like it, are significant in that they mark an important shift toward attempts to substantiate diagnostic labels with neuroscientific findings rather than merely describing a set of behaviors associated with a mental disorder. Approaching DBDs at the level of systemic and organ dysfunction will be a difficult but necessary task, which will help us go beneath the descriptive surface.

4.2.3 SOCIAL FACTORS

Three aspects of social domains impact the development of antisocial and aggressive behavior, and by extension, DBDs—family, peers, and the neighborhood.

Parental engagement in criminal activity is a strong predictor for the development of DBDs. The familial effects likely originate from modeling and compromised parenting of either the permissive or authoritarian or undifferentiated variety. Stressful events, such as separation, divorce, and open conflict in families are all predictive but seem to not have as much impact as parenting style and temperament and their interaction. As youths age into adolescence, familial effects weaken, and peer influences become more important. We next look at some of the most recent relevant studies.

During the course of a 14-year longitudinal study, Barker, Oliver, Viding, Salekin, and Maughan (2011) were the first to examine the impact of maternal prenatal risk factors, fearless temperament, and early parenting on the development of callous–unemotional traits. Youth with conduct problems and callous–unemotional traits were most often the first among their peers to meet formal criteria for conduct disorder. Boys and girls with conduct problems and psychopathic traits were also more likely to have mothers suffering from mental illness, were more likely to have been exposed to harsher parenting practices, and were the recipients of less parental warmth. Among the families looked at in this study, harsh parenting practices directed toward youth with a fearless temperament were a particularly worrisome combination (Barker et al., 2011).

Another important prospective study by Fergusson and Lynskey (1996) looked at the factors predicting resiliency to childhood adversity in a birth cohort of 940 New Zealander youth from birth to age 16. Using a "general index of family adversity" they identified youth who had encountered high levels of family adversity during childhood. Resilient youth were defined as those who lacked a tendency to engage in externalizing behaviors (e.g., absence of substance use, truancy, involvement with law enforcement, conduct and oppositional defiant disorder) in the face of childhood family adversity. This study found that resilient teens tended to engage in less novelty seeking and spend less time with delinquent peers and had higher IQ scores (Fergusson & Lynskey, 1996). In our opinion, this study nicely illustrates the interplay between genetic factors (e.g., temperament), environment (e.g., peer group), and their connection with resilience (e.g., IQ).

While prenatal and genetic factors seem to play a role in the development of conduct problems and callous–unemotional traits in particular, there appear to be differences in the impact of certain risk factors based on sex. Prenatal risk factors seemed to have a more direct effect on the development of conduct problems and psychopathic traits in girls. For boys, prenatal risk factors were associated with fearless temperament and being the receiver of harsh parenting practices. In general, having a fearless temperament appeared to convey the greatest risk of developing conduct problems and callous–unemotional traits.

This study's findings underscore the utility of taking temperament into account when designing interventions for youth with conduct problems and callous–unemotional traits (Fergusson & Lynskey, 1996).

In addition to family, peer influences also effect the etiology of antisocial and aggressive behavior, especially during adolescence. They may be particularly gender specific (Celio, Karnik, & Steiner, 2006). For some youth antisocial behavior and aggression becomes a way of life through affiliation with gangs and other antisocial groups. Such affiliations often substitute for the protective role that family should play. A 2012 study by Van Ryzin and Leve examined the effects hanging out with delinquent peers had on teenage girls taking part in multidimensional treatment foster care (MTFC). MTFC is an effective intervention for delinquent youth that relies on placing them with specially trained foster parents who provide close supervision. MTFC is thought to work in part by preventing young peoples' exposure to the negative influence of delinquent peers that are part and parcel with therapeutic group homes. In this study, MTFC was found to be an effective means of reducing teenage girls' contact with delinquent peers at 12 months, which in turn led to reductions in delinquent behavior at 24 months after the start of MTFC. This study is consistent with earlier studies that attest to the effectiveness of MTFC and underscores the impact that peer affiliation has on DBDs (Van Ryzin & Leve, 2012).

4.2.3.1 Media Effects

The American Academy of Pediatrics released a policy statement in 2009 citing a great deal of evidence on the negative impact that media violence can have on children and teenagers. Violence on television and in video games and violent attitudes in music have been associated with increased levels of physical aggression, increased worries about being the victim of violence, and "desensitization" to violent behavior (American Academy of Pediatrics, 2009).

According to a 2010 meta-analysis by Anderson and colleagues, which included studies from Japan and a variety of Western countries, violent video games carry the potential for leading to a host of problems. Violent video games are apparently a "causal risk factor" for aggressive thinking, aggressive emotional displays or "aggressive affect," and aggressive behavior. Not surprisingly, according to this meta-analysis, violent video games are also associated with reduced empathy and decreased "prosocial" or altruistic behavior. These data were true across sexes and cultural backgrounds (Anderson et al., 2010).

Despite the negative impact violent video games may have on youth, all hope is not lost for video game lovers. Studies involving positive or "prosocial" video games have recently been shown to increase empathy and helping behaviors in young people (Prot et al., 2014). Another recent meta-analysis found that violent video games tend to be associated with increased levels of aggression and reduced prosocial functioning. However, prosocial video games were found to have the opposite effect on young people (Greitemeyer & Mügge, 2014).

In contrast with some of these findings, a recent meta-analysis conducted by Ferguson (2015) suggests that violent video games do not lead to increased aggression, antisocial behavior, poorer academic performance, and/or increased symptoms of mental illness a meaningful way. Ferguson discusses how some academics' personal "anti-game" agendas and publication bias may have led many to overestimate the potentially negative impact of violent video games.

These discrepancies in the literature regarding media influences raise another issue in academic publishing. Briefly stated, it is the tendency for academic journals to cherry-pick the studies they believe their readership will find compelling. For instance, most academic journals do not tend to publish articles with "humdrum" outright negative findings. What is published most often are studies that can lend positive support to and "prove" a given hypothesis. To draw an analogy, publication bias is kind of like watching a movie and editing out all the boring scenes, leaving one with only part of the story. Ferguson (2015) adds that literature on aggression in general may suffer the ill effects of publication bias. While we agree that publication bias is a real issue and think that the findings of this meta-analysis are worth noting, we would advise parents to proceed with caution in letting their children, especially those with disruptive behavior disorders, play violent video games.

What may help greatly in this context is a recommendation issued by the American Academy of Pediatrics in 2014, which was summarized as follows:

> Research has demonstrated a link between screen violence and real-world aggression, both in traditional media like violent movies and in newer media including first-person shooter games. Minimizing exposure to virtual violence will not completely eliminate acts of aggression, but it is an important strategy to investigate. ("The Damaging Effect of Media Violence on Young Children," 2014)

4.2.3.2 Neighborhood Effects

The famous architect Eliel Saarinen once said, "Always design a thing by considering it in its next larger context—a chair in a room, a room in a house, a house in an environment, an environment in a city plan." With Saarinen's comment in mind, we introduce a study published in *JAMA* in 2014 that investigated the influence of housing mobility interventions on adolescents' mental health. The housing interventions in this study were designed to move families out of high-poverty neighborhoods to new homes in low-poverty areas. Many of the boys in this study who moved from high to low poverty areas had significantly higher rates of conduct disorder, PTSD, and depression. In contrast, girls whose families participated in housing mobility interventions seemed to fair better as evidenced by reduced rates of conduct disorder and depression (Kessler et al., 2014). We believe that these data are in line with our belief that disruptive behavior disorders do not fit neatly into the disease model espoused by the DSM-5 but instead represent a variety of conditions that, while sharing similar characteristics, develop in unique biologic, environmental, social, and economic contexts.

4.2.4 PSYCHOPATHY: THE WORST POSSIBLE OUTCOME

The following studies are interesting because they show that it is possible to generate stronger findings when the diagnostic category is narrowed down to a most pernicious variety of DBDs, psychopathy and its correlates such as callous–unemotional traits. Unfortunately, the diagnostic category has been eliminated in the DSM-5. Unlike DBDs and antisocial personality disorder, psychopathy represents a relatively homogenous group of individuals. This makes them interesting for the study of causal factors for at least two reasons: (a) We may develop a deeper understanding of the role of biopsychosocial factors, their relative importance and interplay, and their role in epigenetic development, and (b) in a more pragmatic vein, if we have solid findings regarding causal factors in psychopathy we can intervene and prevent this most pernicious subtype of DBDs, which is a much needed addition to our therapeutic array.

The American author and mythologist Joseph Campbell once wrote, "The folktale is the primer of the picture-language of the soul." Folktales and myths can offer important insights into the commonalities of human experience across cultures and throughout time. A classic German folktale that was immortalized by the Brothers Grimm, "The Story of a Boy Who Went Forth to Learn Fear," seems fitting for this chapter. In this tale, a young boy desperately wants to know fear and is troubled by his inability to "shudder" in response to things that others find terrifying. The boy goes through a variety of trials to learn what fear is including a confrontation with a gravedigger posing as a ghost, a night spent under the gallows with a group of fresh corpses, and three nights in a haunted castle to no avail. Ultimately, it is a bucket of ice-cold water that gives the boy a sense of what it's like for others to "shudder" in fear. Although it is up for debate exactly what message this folktale was originally meant to convey, we next discuss how the young hero it describes shares some characteristics with youth who have psychopathic traits.

Psychopathy can be identified in both children and adults and can be conceptualized as a developmental disorder (Blair, Peschardt, Budhani, Mitchell, & Pine, 2006; Frick, O'Brien, Wootton, & McBurnett, 1994; Hare, 1980; Hare &

Vertommen, 1991). However, Blair and colleagues (2006) point out that one of the missing pieces in our knowledge about psychopathy is the lack of longitudinal studies looking at the likelihood of childhood psychopathy persisting into adulthood. Interestingly, both adults and children with psychopathic traits share common neurocognitive differences that are unlikely to have spontaneously appeared in adulthood.

We now know that as much as 25% of youth and adults with antisocial traits will also display psychopathic traits (Hart & Hare, 1996). A hallmark feature of psychopathic individuals spanning age groups is their facile use of "cold" aggression. This form of aggression, also referred to as PIP, is premeditated and goal directed in its execution. Psychopathic individuals are able to use this type of aggression as a tool to have their needs met. Unlike most of us, psychopathic individuals do not readily associate fear, shame, or remorse with their aggressive antisocial behaviors.

These youth and adults share hallmark character traits (e.g., reduced capacity for empathy and guilt) and behavioral tendencies (e.g., propensity for violence and criminality; Frick et al., 1994; Hare, 1980, 1991; Hare & Vertommen, 1991). Moreover, our current knowledge about the origins of psychopathy suggests that a variety of factors (e.g., genetic, neuroanatomic, cognitive, environmental) affect its development.

In chapters 1 and 2, we introduced the distinction between emotionally charged (RADI) and cold (PIP) antisocial acts and aggression. This distinction should have many implications for the study of psychopathy. As a reminder, "hot" aggression is characterized as occurring in "the heat of the moment" in response to readily identifiable triggers. The hot or RADI form of aggression is well characterized in humans and animals and is associated in a dose-related fashion with our fight-or-flight response. It relies on neuroanatomic structures running between the amygdala to an area of the midbrain referred to as the periaqueductal gray (Gregg & Siegel, 2001; Panksepp, 1998). In contrast to those with psychopathic traits, nonpsychopathic individuals tend to experience guilt, shame, and/or remorse after acts of hot aggression, once they have had an opportunity to cool down.

By contrast, Blair and colleagues (2006) place cold aggression in the domain of goal-directed activity mediated by the same neuroanatomic structures that carry out all other forms of goal-directed activity in the striatum and premotor cortex (Passingham & Toni, 2001; Steiner, 2006). Put another way, cold aggression is carried out at the neuroanatomic level by the same widely distributed brain regions that are responsible for helping one decide whether to walk to the store to buy a pack of gum, whether to withdraw money from a bank account, or whether to cheat on one's tax return. Thus the cold aggression of a psychopathic individual is not a reaction to trauma or perceived threat; rather it represents specific types of instrumental, goal-oriented behavior, coldly calculated and strategized to have needs met (Blair et al., 2006).

While it is common for individuals with psychopathy to display a mixture of both hot and cold aggression, Blair and colleagues (2006) have postulated that there are different neural mechanisms underlying hot aggression in individuals with psychopathic traits. These youth and adults have amygdalae that are less responsive to threat. In other words, these individuals do not scare easily; their hearts do not race when danger is near. Therefore, it is thought that the reactive aggression they display may be due to differences in how their ventrolateral prefrontal cortex is regulated, that is, that these individuals also have a deficit in self-regulation that, among other things, affects the circuitry involved in the threat detection and fight-or-flight response system.

Psychopathic individuals tend to be less responsive to trauma, thus trauma alone is not believed to be the essential ingredient that sends these individuals down the path to psychopathy. Basic genetic, neuroanatomic, and autonomic differences are believed to underlie the cognitive differences observed in psychopathic versus nonpsychopathic individuals. The amygdalae of psychopathic individuals are less responsive to punishment (called "aversive conditioning tasks" in Blair et al., 2006) and to tasks involving emotional learning (Birbaumer et al., 2005; Müller et al., 2003; Veit et al., 2002). Additionally, psychopathic individuals experience less activation of their autonomic nervous system when observing—even on a subliminal level—signs of distress in others. They also have a harder time recognizing fearful facial expressions and speech patterns. Therefore, psychopathic individuals' reduced reactivity to their personal experience of traumatic events, their dampened responses to the unfortunate plight of others, and an impaired ability to even recognize distress in others make it difficult for a social-emotional construct like empathy to take root. Empathy induction, on the other hand, is the most effective way parents use to have children desist from being antisocial and aggressive toward others. If this self-regulation system is defunct—as it seems to be in psychopathy—it will be very difficult to socialize children's antisocial and aggressive behavior, as Aichhorn (1935) has suggested is necessary, in order to encourage them to use aggression in an adaptive fashion and to treat full-fledged psychopathy once it has emerged.

4.2.4.1 Biological Factors in Psychopathy

For decades, the scientific community has been aware that people with psychopathic personalities and career criminals have differences in fear conditioning and baseline arousal in many different channels (heart rate, galvanic skin response, EEG, hormonal) relative to the general population (Hare, 1978). Such differences were first proposed and studied by Hans Eysenck in the UK, resulting in interesting leads, which were mostly confirmed in his seminal studies in *Crime and Personality* (1964) and later editions (Eysenck & Eysenck, 1970).

These findings were further elaborated on by Adrian Raine (2013), among others, as summarized in his book, *The Psychopathology of Crime*. In his book, Raine makes a very strong case to look at criminal activity from a psychiatric clinical point of view.

Since then, there has been a steady accrual of evidence that helps us identify this aberrant developmental trajectory rooted in neurodevelopmental differences. Raine's (2013) crucial prospective follow-up of a birth cohort in Madagascar from infancy to adulthood provided strong evidence for the link between low arousal and future antisocial and aggressive behavior. Although subsequently not all studies have confirmed these findings, because of the strong design of this lengthy follow-up study the results still must be considered as very relevant today.

Taking the deficient arousal findings directly to the brain structures involved in generating emotional arousal, Marsh and colleagues (2008) were among the first to investigate amygdala activation in youth with behavior problems and callous–unemotional traits. Additionally, they were the first to examine the neuroanatomic similarities and differences between youth with callous–unemotional traits and ADHD. What they found was that young people with callous–unemotional traits displayed reductions in amygdala activation in response to observing fearful facial expressions relative to controls and youth with a diagnosis of ADHD. Observations from this study indicate that youth with callous–unemotional traits may have reduced connectivity between their amygdala and ventromedial prefrontal cortex relative to children with ADHD and controls. This was an important study because it was the first indication that youth with callous–unemotional traits have reduced amygdala activation in response to observing distress in others (Marsh et al., 2008).

White and colleagues' (2012) findings are consistent with previous research showing that youth with psychopathic traits have reduced amygdala activation as observed via fMRI in response to observing distress in others. Participants were shown faces with either fearful or neutral expressions on a computer screen. Adjacent to the face on each side were digital bars that varied on a continuum from between being parallel with one another to intersecting at 90-degree angles, and participants were tasked with commenting on whether they were parallel. When the bars were parallel or nearly parallel (i.e., the "high attentional load" condition) participants needed to recruit more cognitive resources to determine whether the bars were parallel versus when the bars where clearly not parallel (i.e., the "low attentional load" condition). In this experiment the amygdalae of controls and youth with psychopathic traits did not differ in response to neutral versus fearful facial expressions under the high attentional load condition.

However, when the bars were obviously not parallel with one another in the low attentional load condition, youth with psychopathic traits showed a markedly reduced activation of their amygdalae when the task was paired with a fearful facial expression as compared controls who showed marked activation of their amygdalae. One could reasonably argue that the youth in this study with disruptive behavior disorders and psychopathic traits had simply learned to avoid paying attention to fearful facial expressions, but through the fMRI, such a hypothesis was laid to rest. The fMRI data of participants with disruptive behavior disorders and psychopathic traits indicated that they did not recruit brain regions associated with top-down attentional control when exposed to fearful facial expressions under the low attentional load condition. In other words, the fMRI findings suggested that the lack of response to fearful facial expressions observed in children with disruptive behavior disorders and psychopathic traits was not due to the intentional avoidance of emotional stimuli. Rather, those with disruptive behavior disorders and accompanying psychopathic traits seem to possess fundamental differences in how they process the emotional expressions of others (White et al., 2012).

While the findings of this last study are thought-provoking, it is good to remind ourselves of some important limitations of imaging studies like the one by White and colleagues (2012). The study had too few participants, and the gender distribution was skewed in a manner that made it difficult to draw firm conclusions. For instance, it is possible that the increased proportion of girls in the control group may have skewed the results in favor of the study's conclusion that youth with disruptive behavior disorders and accompanying psychopathic traits tend to respond less robustly to the emotional distress of others. Also, the youth in this study were between the ages of 10 and 17, which means that there had been plenty of time for life events (e.g., incidents of physical and/or emotional trauma, heavy substance abuse) to substantially alter their developmental trajectories. A replication study with a larger and younger sample size would be ideal for determining if the differences observed were due to some form of genetic deficit. Despite the limitations described, this study has important implications for our understanding of psychopathy, as it was among the first neuroimaging studies involving children with psychopathic traits.

Fortunately, an additional recent neuroimaging study had findings consistent with earlier findings regarding amygdala activation in youth with callous–unemotional traits. Youth with callous–unemotional traits showed diminished amygdala reactivity when observing emotional distress in others. Difficulties empathizing with others have been postulated as a fundamental ingredient for cold aggression (Lozier, Cardinale, VanMeter, & Marsh, 2014).

Additional research has looked at the biologic and hormonal underpinnings of psychopathic personality traits in youth. One such study investigated the link between hypothalamic pituitary adrenal (HPA) axis reactivity and aggression in boys with ADHD who also displayed symptoms of disruptive behavior disorders. The boys in this study with a high degree of callous–unemotional traits were shown to have more behavioral problems and a diminished reactivity of their HPA axis. In contrast, the boys with ADHD who did not have concomitant callous–unemotional traits tended to have fewer behavior problems and did not have a blunted HPA reactivity in response to stress (Stadler et al., 2011).

There is a growing body of literature correlating widely distributed abnormalities in brain structure and function with antisocial behavior in adolescents. Rather than discrete areas of dysfunction, recent literature suggests problems in multiple interconnected brain regions (e.g., dorsomedial orbitofrontal, prefrontal, limbic system) that are involved with the handing of emotions (Raschle, Menks, Fehlbaum, Tshomba, & Stadler, 2015).

A recent study provided a rare longitudinal glimpse at some of the neurobiological correlates of aggression. Levels of hot and cold aggression were assessed among a sample of boys and girls at ages 10, 12, 15, and 18. At the age of 18 the authors collected data on skin conductance fear conditioning. Their results were consistent with previous studies showing that individuals with a propensity for cold aggression tend to have a diminished conditioned fear response. Hot aggression, on the other hand, was not associated with reduced autonomic arousal (Gao, Tuvblad, Schell, Baker, & Raine, 2015).

In sum, the basic science investigation of callous–unemotional traits and psychopathy is beginning to connect with the earlier literature on peripheral arousal deficits producing findings that are in line with the Eysenck/Raine hypotheses. However, we still need more clarity of the early manifestations of these deficits through imaging techniques, eliminating the effects of years of malnutrition, abuse, head trauma, drug abuse, and alcohol abuse. In psychopathy, we are still in the position that these basic science findings are interesting but not ready for clinical application.

4.2.4.2 *Psychological Factors in Psychopathy*

Gao et al. (2010) pursued the specific question of associations of fear conditioning and antisocial and aggressive behavior further. The authors set about to look at the impact of differences in electrodermal fear conditioning on the development of both aggressive and nonaggressive forms of antisocial behavior among boys and girls. What they discovered was that less aggressive boys and girls in this study responded more readily to fear conditioning. Also, the better the fear conditioning between ages three and eight, the less aggression observed at age eight in both boys and girls. However, this distinction was less clear with nonviolent forms of aggression. This study showed how differences in fear conditioning, most likely related to neurodevelopmental abnormalities in the amygdala, have downstream effects on children's risk of committing violent acts. This study expands the relevance of the Eysenck/Raine hypotheses to both genders, adding an important developmental trajectory from infancy to school age. They also link to the important literature on parenting and the influences of abuse and temperament on the prosocial adjustment of individuals at high risk for adverse outcomes of antisocial behavior and aggression (Gao, Raine, Venables, Dawson, & Mednick, 2010).

Deficits in affective perspective-taking abilities (i.e., empathizing with others) have been hypothesized as a contributing factor to conduct problems in youth (Jones, Happé, Gilbert, Burnett, & Viding, 2010). One creatively designed study addressing this issue contrasted the cognitive and affective perspective-taking abilities of children with conduct disorder versus healthy controls. In this study, children with conduct disorder with a relatively low degree of callous–unemotional traits had problems in both cognitive and emotional perspective taking. However, children in this study with a high degree of callous–unemotional traits tended to have intact cognitive perspective-taking abilities with deficits in affective perspective taking. In other words, according to this study, youth with callous–unemotional traits are well able to place themselves "in the shoes" of others on an intellectual level yet are not facile in their ability to identify with others on an emotional level. These findings helped to point out the heterogeneity among youth with conduct disorder, made a case for subtyping youth with callous–unemotional traits, underscored the need for more individualized treatment approaches for youth with conduct disorder, and helped lay the groundwork for investigating the variety of developmental pathways leading to hot and cold forms of aggression. Of note, this study's subjects primarily consisted of boys, so it is unclear whether its findings are applicable to girls (Anastassiou-Hadjicharalambous & Warden, 2008).

A recent study (Ueno & Schwenck, 2015) looked at differences in both cognitive and affective perspective taking in girls with conduct problems with and without callous–unemotional traits as compared to healthy controls. In contrast to the previously discussed study (Anastassiou-Hadjicharalambous & Warden, 2008), there were no differences in perspective-taking ability between the three groups. We contend that the differences between the two studies we have just described calls attention to the wide-ranging variables and variety of developmental pathways involved in the emergence of conduct problems and callous–unemotional traits.

Sterzer and Stadler (2009) published one of the early review articles focused on neuroimaging's ability to identify some of the functional and structural correlates of conduct problems in youth. They described how differences in information processing in social settings is associated with conduct problems, as Dodge's group has repeatedly reported in his behaviorally based studies, which are now beginning to be replicated in many different countries and continents (Dodge et al., 2015; Sterzer & Stadler, 2009). Sterzer and Stadler additionally found that youth with conduct problems have differences in the self-regulation of social and goal-directed behaviors. For instance, these youth were shown to have structural abnormalities associated with difficulties in recognizing emotions (e.g., amygdala), emotion regulation (e.g., orbito-frontal cortex), reinforcement learning (e.g., ventromedial prefrontal cortex), cognitive control (e.g., anterior cingulate gyrus), and performance monitoring (e.g., temporo-parietal cortex), once again extending their behavioral observations into highly relevant brain systems and subsystems.

We have long appreciated the contribution certain adverse child characteristics (temperament, attachment status) can make to deviant development and adverse parenting. A recent meta-analysis adds considerable support to the idea that certain characteristics of children make them more or less sensitive to parenting, as well as highlighting what underlying psychological characteristics contribute to producing this effect. Difficult temperament, as constituted by negative emotionality, and trouble with effortful control were significantly more vulnerable to negative parenting but also benefitted more from positive parenting. Effortful control did not consistently moderate associations between parenting and the adjustment of the child. The strongest associations were found in studies that used observed behaviors rather than self-report for both parenting and child adjustment. Many of the findings were based on prospective follow-up studies (Slagt, Dubas, Deković, & van Aken, 2016).

These current psychological studies continue to be more proximal to clinical practice than the biological studies previously mentioned. They hold great promise to design specific intervention packages targeting, in a concerted fashion, the areas implicated in antisocial and aggressive behaviors that have strong links to very pernicious outcomes.

4.3 Implications for Clinical Practice

We are now ready to examine the impact the etiological mosaic we have discussed has on clinical practice. Retaining the tripartite division of the biopsychosocial model in psychiatry, we find that there is much recent research (originating between 2011 and 2016) that is pertinent and of improving quality supporting the relevance of all three factors in the study of DBDs. The most promising new leads come from genetic and imaging studies; in addition, there are many studies that add to the weight of previously existing psychological and social studies. But to date, there are no true breakthrough studies, except perhaps in the subdomain of psychopathy and its psychological correlates.

Similar to many other diagnoses in the DSM or ICD identifying psychopathology, we find that our current stage of knowledge is such that we have basically no definitive data identifying etiologies in the DBD group. This should come as no surprise. As we discussed in chapters 2 and 3, the current diagnoses are broadly based, nonexclusive, and of unknown validity. The theoretical stance of the DSM and ICD system, which discourages thinking about pathogenetic processes in order to preserve a theoretically unbiased stance, essentially would lead to such a state of affairs. It is true that in all sciences knowledge starts with careful surface observation and classification, but it should not stop there if true progress is to be achieved. One goes beneath the surface and looks for causal processes, be they biological, psychological, or social, some combination thereof, or rationally reduced to the most important one by a careful scientific process. The DSM and ICD are stuck in a process of description and redescription and grouping and regrouping based on data that are not able to lead us in the most relevant direction. As we have suggested, developmental psychopathology as a theory and developmental psychiatry as an application of this theory hold much greater promise in the area of DBDs to resolve many issues for the clinician. As we discussed in chapter 2, the National Institute of Mental Health's departure from using the DSM as a research tool relegates the system to one of clinical application. As such, it may have some helpful functionality; although, as we mentioned in chapter 2, a recent and informal poll of psychiatric practitioners found that less than 10% in fact use the DSM as a guiding system in their practice, which also calls that into question. It may well be that the ICD and DSM are relegated in the final analysis to an insurance coding system, unless there is more substantive work done, at least as far as DBDs are concerned.

A clinician or researcher should look for in an etiology is a well-established causal chain that connects the genotype of a disorder (if that is relevant) to the phenotype—that is, the external observable manifestations in the consulting room. This allows for decisions to be made about how to target each link in the causal chain specifically to disruptive disorders and potentially heal the disease. The best established model for etiology derives from the Koch experiments regarding the etiology of bacterial disease. Unfortunately, this model does not help much in psychopathology and in DBDs in particular.

In the DBD domain, we must deal with the fact that problems with antisocial and aggressive behavior are of heterogeneous etiological origin. Figure 4.3 demonstrates this state of affairs.

Figure 4.3 summarizes the possible psychiatric diagnoses, which in the literature have been shown to be correlated with (not necessarily the cause of) problems with antisocial behavior and aggression. These diagnoses range from central nervous system (CNS) injury and trauma, an exogenous event, to

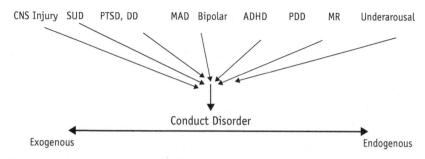

Figure 4.3 The current CD label: A final common pathway.

intellectual disabilities and callous–unemotional traits, which are presumably predominantly endogenously driven (by, e.g. genetic transmission). ADHD and PTSD are sandwiched in the middle, because as far as we know we can think of them as disorders with a substantial genetic predisposition that are precipitated by some promotor event (i.e., traumatic exposure in the case of PTSD).

The ideal study that would help us define the etiology of problems with antisocial behavior and aggression would take its pointers from a great deal of convergent evidence from epidemiological studies, which then leads to studies of specific targets of endogenous mechanisms linking genotype to phenotype, decisively confirming the causal role of some of these mechanisms in the pathogenesis of DBDs. These mechanisms would then be manipulated in laboratory experiments with high internal validity, that is, as much error-free design as possible. A series of clinical studies with specific treatments targeting these causal mechanisms would close this loop. Results presumably would show that as these causal mechanisms are disrupted or even repaired, the disorder would recede and be healed.

In reviewing the evidence in chapter 3 and the relevant studies in this chapter, we can see immediately that this is not the status of research in DBDs. Most of the information necessary to complete these lines of investigation are missing. We have interesting leads and strong hunches but no error-proof facts. Upon further reflection, we immediately can see that DBDs are not the exception in the realm of psychiatry and psychopathology. It can reasonably be argued that psychiatrists and neuroscientists encounter complexities in studying and treating psychopathology unlike most other fields in medicine. So it is little wonder that there always have been and still are movements underfoot to reduce complex disorders, such as DBDs to a biological substrate in hopes of gaining respectability in medicine (we are doctors too). We argue that this is a prematurely orthodox stance, which serves no one well—patients, their doctors, or neuroscientists.

Having acknowledged the difficulties we are encountering in DBDs where we have evidence for biopsychosocial candidates for causality, we will be better off, in an interim step, to construct a theoretical model that accommodates multiple causal factors from biology, psychology, and sociology to be comprehensive and correct. Figure 4.4 summarizes this model in schematic form.

Figure 4.4 shows what our data so far suggest. DBDs are syndromes of a dysfunctional CNS, a very complex biological machine that through some barely understood mechanisms generates an entity we call mind. Both CNS and mind are surrounded by social environments, which can be very intimate (as in primary caregiver and family) or distant (as in schools, neighborhoods, communities). The evidence we have at the present points to the fact that there are multiple bottom-up and top-down causal influences. The size of the arrows suggests the power of the causal loop. The CNS causes the mind in a bottom-up causal loop, but we also know that the mind can cause alterations in brain functioning. The mind will look for social environments that map closely on its appetites and expectancies. For example, youth with drug addiction will very often try to associate with peer groups that practice and cherish drug use. That in turn will result in a top-down causal loop: because drugs are valued in this particular culture, individuals will not be very motivated to resist drug use. They may seek to enhance their social status in this particular social world by acquiring, selling, and providing drugs for the group. These activities may then, in fact, lead to an alteration in the brain's hedonic set point to where it becomes increasingly impossible for biological reasons to cease drug use and desist from antisocial activities associated with the acquisition and sale of the drugs, such as owning a weapon, getting into fights, and so on.

Similar scenarios can be constructed for the use of aggression and violence in an instrumental, calculated way to achieve one's goals, for example, for theft of goods to provide a family and friends with needed supplies and materials.

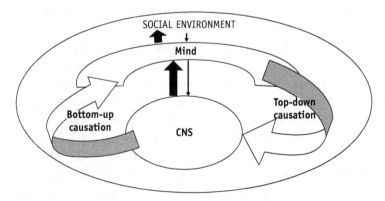

Figure 4.4 The comprehensive biopsychosocial model of DBDs.

From this model, we can see immediately how the clinician needs to be mindful of all these factors. At the present time we do not know which one of these loops is the most important to disrupt. In most cases it will be clinically prudent to attack all of them: disrupt dyssocial peer contacts, make abstinence a goal to achieve in either outpatient of elevated care settings, build the individual's ability to resist cravings by giving drugs such as Neurontin, and hopefully at some point in the not too distant future correct or neutralize the genetic predispositions that facilitate emergence of disorders when a precipitating causal factor is added to the mix.

We next present specific cases that demonstrate the causal loops originating from the CNS, the mind, and the social environment.

Case 1 illustrates the powerful influence of peers (the social environment) on vulnerable youth. Arturo was part of recent immigrant family from Mexico. The family moved to the United States one year prior to the events that brought him to the attention of the school and police. While his English was steadily improving, Arturo still struggled with the academic demands. Attending a predominantly white and Asian school, he was not tied in with any particular group, although he was very keen on being part of one. Thus when one of the more prominent white peers invited him to be part of "a school farm raid," he happily agreed. Four boys broke and entered the school on the weekend and killed dozens of chickens that were kept in a special enclosure. As a function of this raid, Arturo's standing rose considerably at school. He was part of the inner circle. Demands on him to perform more antisocial acts did not stop. The same group of boys revisited the school on several occasions to continue to vandalize the place, at one point pouring cement in many of the classroom locks. They were caught on video and arrested. Examining Arturo's background, it turned out that his mother had advanced cancer that responded poorly to treatment. She was incapacitated much of the time. Since money was a serious issue, his mother also dropped her chemotherapy for her cancer, knowing that this would put her life in jeopardy. In addition, as his mother had to quit her job, Arturos's father started working two shifts in a warehouse, sometimes even three to help the family make ends meet. The net effect was that Arturo received little or no supervision and guidance. There were no other risk factors for his conduct disorder of biological or psychological nature.

Case 2 demonstrates the influence of psychological variables in the development of severe conduct problems leading to episodes of hot aggression. A 16-year-old white male, Glen, was convicted of manslaughter. He was examined after adjudication and during serving his sentence, so there was very little incentive for him to try to exculpate his actions by faking psychopathology. The youth had attempted together with a friend to steal a car radio from a new truck in a convenience store parking lot. As they attempted to remove the radio, the owner of the truck returned. Realizing what was happening, the owner started scream-ing abuse and storming across the parking lot to the truck. The youth froze, una-ble to move, holding his tools in his hand. The closer the irate man came, the more scared the youth became, and he was convinced that the man was going to kill him. He thought he saw a knife in the man's hand. Anticipating his own demise, the youth struck the man with the screwdriver in the neck, causing lethal injury. While this was occurring, he did not remember having any other ideas as to how to settle this situation. It never occurred to him to run away, talk the man down, offer to fix the damage, make up some story about why he wanted the radio, and so on. This extreme psychological narrowing of choices in conflictual situations has been shown to be one of the most powerful accompaniments of conduct disorders. The youth clearly knew he was doing wrong by stealing the radio and striking the man. He did not attempt to run away after the crime; he just sat down next to the dying man waiting for the police, called by witnesses to come and pick him up. He was devastated that the truck owner never was found to have a weapon on himself. He was convinced he saw a knife in the owner's hand as he approached. He knew he had done wrong, readily owned up to his crime, and began significant therapeutic work to change his perceptions. He was described by his parents as a fearful child who would readily go along with anti-social exploits out of fear that he would be retaliated against if he did not. The neighborhood he grew up in lacked structure and was crime infested. Orienting toward its antisocial values was part of having to survive in it. This is a typical case of Eysenck's anxious pathway into crime: in the right social context, anxiety becomes a risk, not a protective factor. The crime also is a good illustration of the dose-responsive character of RADI aggression: the closer the furious truck owner came, the greater the real and perceived threat became. Flight was impos-sible, so it turned into fight. The rapidity of this progression suggests that this threat detection system was primed by living for years in a threatening and even dangerous environment.

Case 3 is a case of a cold-blooded killer. This is the case of a 17-year-old male, Ted, who was apprehended after killing three men at the banks of a river in southern California. The men were three homeless people who fished for food in the river. The perpetrator had noticed them for some time being "on his terri-tory." Once he had pistol whipped them in order to scare them away. However, because this seemed to be a lucky fishing spot, the three men kept returning for more fish. The youth then observed their patterns of behavior for a while, notic-ing that they would consume large amounts of beer and marihuana during the day to the point of almost complete inebriation by late afternoon. This was also the time when there were very few people down by the river, thus chances were he would be unobserved. He then went down to the banks of the river and shot all three men execution style. When asked why he committed these crimes, he hissed disdainfully: "they were in my face, man!" shaking his head in disbelief that he even needed to explain that. His resting heart rate was 56 BPM; he had an extreme callous–unemotional score. He refused to do any other psychometrics, saying he did not give a damn and he knew he had to be let go at 25 anyway. Prior to this crime, he had a long history of stealing cars, driving them extremely fast and carelessly in a residential area, instigating gang-related fights, organizing drug purchase and sales where he would often cheat the parties involved, challenging his gang friends to playing chicken or Russian roulette—all of these events were undetected, never reported by his parents as much as they were aware of them at all and never adjudicated. His mother was a heroin-addicted prostitute. His father was a contract killer for one of the local gangs currently in a trial regarding his latest killing. The youth would describe him admiringly as "a cool dude—nobody messes with him." The youth himself had risen very high in his own gang and had plans to be top boss. This case illustrates the pernicious power of biological predilection in the context of active and reinforcing modelling of cold aggression and predation. This young man was well on his way to psychopathy as a long-term outcome.

Case 4 examines interaction between difficult temperament and negative parenting (constitution and social factors). This case involves a four-year-old girl referred for evaluation as a result of being asked to leave her kindergarten. This was the third time in the span of six months. She was ejected because of her temper tantrums in response to many of the teacher's demands—to stay in line, to be seated, to listen to a story, to sit quietly and draw. In addition, she would often get in fights with other children over sharing toys. She would sulk for long periods of time when disciplined. She would not accept any time-outs, arguing vociferously that the other person involved in an event always was in the wrong. When calm and cooperative, she was able to perform many cognitive tasks ahead of expectations (writing her name, counting to 100, etc.). Her mother was a single woman with a long history of depression and intermittent alcoholism. When the child's pediatric record was reviewed, it showed that she had reached all milestones on time, some—like speech—even precociously. Her temperament was assessed as difficult at age 1.6 years: she was very active and had mostly negative affect. Her sleep and feeding schedules were always irregular. Of note, her mother requested an evaluation for adoption because the child allegedly deliberately tried to poke her in the eye while she fed her a meal. The mother was told that such planning was simply not possible for a one and a half year old. The mother then elaborated that she had to beat the child repeatedly to stop the child's attacks on her. At this point, child protective services were called in. The mother tearfully insisted on keeping her daughter, promising to stop beating her. It was decided that the mother would be enrolled in parenting classes and the child would remain at home. There was no further follow-up by child protective services, and the mother dropped out of the classes after two months. The pediatric record in the next two years documented very harsh parenting, bordering on abuse. A referral for mental health treatment was not followed. The mother would insist that her daughter brought on this harsh parenting herself because she would not follow simple verbal commands. "She makes me so mad, she is just so stubborn, what else can I do but slap her to stop her from what she is doing? If I don't do it now, she will turn into a criminal."

Case 5 illustrates the power of disrupted attachment and traumatic events, with gang life as a solution. This is the case of a young man, LaVande, who participated as a driver in a gang-related drug deal gone wrong where another gang member who had stolen gang property was executed in an alley. The young man, now 22, was threatened by the death penalty for his participation. A detailed review of his early pediatric, developmental, and criminal record was conducted, along with interviews in prison. The child was born to a 14-year-old teen who was raped. She gave the child up for adoption. He was placed in a series of foster homes until an adoptive parent would become available. This did not come to pass until the child was 3.6 years old, at which point he had been placed in the care of five different homes. Parenthetically, reports by successive placements begin to comment on his increasing emotional distance from staff, other children in the homes, and classmates. He also seemed increasingly irritable and less fun to be with. His adoptive parents were an elderly couple that wanted to do "the parenting we never did" because they never had any children. After two years, they asked the adoption agency to take the boy back, citing, "He is too much of a handful." Pediatric records showed that he was uneven in his development but reached milestones mostly on time. He was somewhat erratic in his circadian rhythmicity but still of a sweet disposition and quite responsive to attention and affection. He did not do well with disappointment, becoming demanding and onerous. Returning into the foster system, he again experienced several placements in the span of three years. At age nine another adoptive parent was found. This parent was a single elementary school teacher living in San Francisco, who already had adopted an 11-year-old boy. This older boy was not happy with LaVande's arrival and seemed to think of him more as a rival than a brother. LaVande developed behavior problems at school with focus, aggression, and getting into fights. He was referred back to his pediatrician who started stimulant treatment for ADHD. It had very little beneficial effects. A referral to child psychiatry was made. In the course of the evaluation, it was found that starting almost immediately after his adoption by the teacher, LaVande was being sexually abused on an almost daily basis by both the teacher and his adoptive brother, sometimes in a threesome, sometimes with just one of them while the other one was taking pictures and movies of the sexual interactions. LaVande, now almost 12, was placed again into a foster home. After one year, his biological mother attempted to make contact with him. She wanted to meet him and seek his understanding for what she had done. He declined to meet her, saying he was not interested in any contact with her. He was placed in a new home because he was found to be using drugs and alcohol on a regular basis. Finally, he was committed to the youth authority for possession and sales at age 14.6. While in the youth authority he joined the Crips who seemed supportive, interested in his welfare, ready to protect him as necessary, and very happy to help him refine his drug sale skills. He was particularly happy to meet Thunder, the local crime boss, who visited his son in the authority regularly. He was offered an important territory after his release that also would allow him to continue work with many of the youngsters in the gang he had come to know and appreciate while incarcerated. Upon hearing of his past travails, the gang had generously offered to have him join without going through all the violent hazings that were quite the norm as an admission ticket. They did not waive the requirement that he needed to kill or be helpful in killing someone who had disrespected the gang or was a snitch. LaVande considered himself special and lucky to be able to fulfill this requirement later on by participating as a driver for the gang members from and to the execution site. Needless to say, he did not report the crime. During the examination before the death penalty hearing, LaVande shrugged his shoulders when he was told that in a best-case scenario, he would not be executed but be sentenced to life without the possibility of parole, to be served in a maximum security prison. His only request was that the psychiatric report on him not include the fact that his rapists and molesters in the adoptive home assaulted him in a homosexual fashion. "I am going to be with a lot of men for the rest of my life and I want to keep it simple."

References

Aichhorn, A. (1935). *Wayward Youth (1925)*. New York, Viking.

American Academy of Pediatrics. (2009). Policy statement—media violence. *Pediatrics, 124*(5), 1495–1503.

Anastassiou-Hadjicharalambous, X., & Warden, D. (2008). Cognitive and affective perspective-taking in conduct-disordered children high and low on callous-unemotional traits. *Child and Adolescent Psychiatry and Mental Health, 2*(1), 16.

Anderson, C. A., Shibuya, A., Ihori, N., Swing, E. L., Bushman, B. J., Sakamoto, A., . . . Saleem, M. (2010). Violent video game effects on aggression, empathy, and prosocial behavior in Eastern and Western countries: A meta-analytic review. *Psychological Bulletin, 136*(2), 151–173.

Baker, L., & Cantwell, D. P. (1987). Factors associated with the development of psychiatric illness in children with early speech/language problems. *Journal of Autism and Developmental Disorders, 17*(4), 499–510.

Barker, E. D., Oliver, B. R., Viding, E., Salekin, R. T., & Maughan, B. (2011). The impact of prenatal maternal risk, fearless temperament and early parenting on adolescent callous-unemotional traits: A 14-year longitudinal investigation. *Journal of Child Psychology and Psychiatry, 52*(8), 878–888.

Beitchman, J. H., Zai, C. C., Muir, K., Berall, L., Nowrouzi, B., Choi, E., & Kennedy, J. L. (2012). Childhood aggression, callous-unemotional traits and oxytocin genes. *European Child & Adolescent Psychiatry, 21*(3), 125–132.

Birbaumer, N., Veit, R., Lotze, M., Erb, M., Hermann, C., Grodd, W., & Flor, H. (2005). Deficient fear conditioning in psychopathy: A functional magnetic resonance imaging study. *Archives of General Psychiatry, 62*(7), 799–805.

Blair, R. J. R., Leibenluft, E., & Pine, D. S. (2014). Conduct disorder and callous–unemotional traits in youth. *The New England Journal of Medicine, 371,* 2207–2216.

Blair, R. J. R., Peschardt, K., Budhani, S., Mitchell, D., & Pine, D. (2006). The development of psychopathy. *Journal of Child Psychology and Psychiatry, 47*(3–4), 262–276.

Bowlby, J. (1946). *Forty-four juvenile thieves: Their characters and home-life.* London: Baillière, Tindall & Cox.

Breslau, N., Lucia, V. C., & Alvarado, G. F. (2006). Intelligence and other predisposing factors in exposure to trauma and posttraumatic stress disorder: A follow-up study at age 17 years. *Archives of General Psychiatry, 63*(11), 1238–1245.

Brier, N. (2001). The relationship between learning disability and delinquency: A review and reappraisal. *Journal of Learning Disabilities, 22*(9), 546–553.

Bronfenbrenner, U. (1986). Ecology of the family as a context for human development: Research perspectives. *Developmental Psychology, 22,* 723–742. doi:10.1037/0012-1649.22.6.723.

Caspi, A., & Moffitt, T. E. (2006). Gene-environment interactions in psychiatry: Joining forces with neuroscience. *Nature Reviews Neuroscience, 7*(7), 583–590.

Caspi, A., Sugden, K., Moffitt, T. E., Taylor, A., Craig, I. W., Harrington, H., ... Poulton, R. (2003). Influence of life stress on depression: Moderation by a polymorphism in the 5-HTT gene. *Science, 301*(5631), 386–389.

Celio, M., Karnik, N. S., & Steiner, H. (2006). Early maturation as a risk factor for aggression and delinquency in adolescent girls: A review. *International Journal of Clinical Practice, 60*(10), 1254–1262.

Cohn, M. D., van Lith, K., Kindt, M., Pape, L. E., Doreleijers, T. A., van den Brink, W., ... Popma, A. (2015). Fear extinction, persistent disruptive behavior and psychopathic traits: fMRI in late adolescence. *Social Cognitive and Affective Neuroscience, 11*(7), 1027–1035.

Dadds, M. R., Moul, C., Cauchi, A., Dobson-Stone, C., Hawes, D. J., Brennan, J., & Ebstein, R. E. (2014). Methylation of the oxytocin receptor gene and oxytocin blood levels in the development of psychopathy. *Development and Psychopathology, 26*(1), 33–40.

Dadds, M. R., Moul, C., Cauchi, A., Dobson-Stone, C., Hawes, D. J., Brennan, J., ... Ebstein, R. E. (2014). Polymorphisms in the oxytocin receptor gene are associated with the development of psychopathy. *Development and Psychopathology, 26*(1), 21–31.

Dodge, K. A., Malone, P. S., Lansford, J. E., Sorbring, E., Skinner, A. T., Tapanya, S., ... Al-Hassan, S. M. (2015). Hostile attributional bias and aggressive behavior in global context. *Proceedings of the National Academy of Sciences, 112*(30), 9310–9315.

Eysenck, H. J. (1964). *Crime and Personality.* Methuen, London.

Eysenck, S. B., & Eysenck, H. J. (1970). Crime and personality: An empirical study of the three-factor theory. *British Journal of Criminology, 10*(3), 225–239.

Ferguson, C. J. (2015). Do Angry Birds make for angry children? A meta-analysis of video game influences on children's and adolescents' aggression, mental health, prosocial behavior, and academic performance. *Perspectives on Psychological Science, 10*(5), 646–666.

Fergusson, D. M., & Lynskey, M. T. (1996). Adolescent resiliency to family adversity. *Journal of Child Psychology and Psychiatry, 37*(3), 281–292.

Frick, P. J., O'Brien, B. S., Wootton, J. M., & McBurnett, K. (1994). Psychopathy and conduct problems in children. *Journal of Abnormal Psychology, 103*(4), 700–707.

Gao, Y., Raine, A., Venables, P. H., Dawson, M. E., & Mednick, S. A. (2010). Reduced electrodermal fear conditioning from ages 3 to 8 years is associated with aggressive behavior at age 8 years. *Journal of Child Psychology and Psychiatry, 51*(5), 550–558.

Gao, Y., Tuvblad, C., Schell, A., Baker, L., & Raine, A. (2015). Skin conductance fear conditioning impairments and aggression: A longitudinal study. *Psychophysiology, 52*(2), 288–295.

Gregg, T. R., & Siegel, A. (2001). Brain structures and neurotansmitters regulating aggression in cats: Implications for human aggression. *Progress in Neuro-Psychopharmacology and Biological Psychiatry, 25*(1), 91–140.

Greitemeyer, T., & Mügge, D. O. (2014). Video games do affect social outcomes: A meta-analytic review of the effects of violent and prosocial video game play. *Personality and Social Psychology Bulletin, 40*(5), 578–589.

Grigorenko, E. L. (2006). Learning disabilities in juvenile offenders. *Child & Adolescent Psychiatry Clinics of North America, 15*(2), 353–371.

Grossman, A. W., Churchill, J. D., McKinney, B. C., Kodish, I. M., Otte, S. L., & Greenough, W. T. (2003). Experience effects on brain development: Possible contributions to psychopathology. *Journal of Child Psychology and Psychiatry, 44*(1), 33–63.

Halperin, J. M., & McKay, K. E. (1998). Psychological testing for child and adolescent psychiatrists: A review of the past 10 years. *Journal of the American Academy for Child & Adolescent Psychiatry, 37*(6), 575–584.

Hare, R. D. (1978). Electrodermal and cardiovascular correlates of psychopathy. In R. D. Hare & D. Schalling (Eds.), *Psychopathic behavior: Approaches to research* (pp. 107–143). Chichester, UK: Wiley.

Hare, R. D. (1980). A research scale for the assessment of psychopathy in criminal populations. *Personality and Individual Differences, 1*(2), 111–119.

Hare, R. D., & Vertommen, H. (1991). *The Hare Psychopathy Checklist–Revised.* North Tonawanda, NY: Multi-Health Systems.

Hart, S. D., & Hare, R. D. (1996). Psychopathy and antisocial personality disorder. *Current Opinion in Psychiatry, 9*(2), 129–132.

Hawes, D. J., & Dadds, M. R. (2005). The treatment of conduct problems in children with callous-unemotional traits. *Journal of Consulting and Clinical Psychology, 73*(4), 737–741.

Hawes, D. J., Price, M. J., & Dadds, M. R. (2014). Callous-unemotional traits and the treatment of conduct problems in childhood and adolescence: A comprehensive review. *Clinical Child and Family Psychology Review, 17*(3), 248–267.

Jones, A. P., Happé, F. G., Gilbert, F., Burnett, S., & Viding, E. (2010). Feeling, caring, knowing: Different types of empathy deficit in boys with psychopathic tendencies and autism spectrum disorder. *Journal of Child Psychology and Psychiatry, 51*(11), 1188–1197.

Kaufman, J., Yang, B. Z., Douglas-Palumberi, H., Grasso, D., Lipschitz, D., Houshyar, S., . . . Gelernter, J. (2006). Brain-derived neurotrophic factor-5-HTTLPR gene interactions and environmental modifiers of depression in children. *Biological Psychiatry, 59*(8), 673–680.

Kavale, K. A., & Forness, S. R. (2000). What definitions of learning disability say and don't say: A critical analysis. *Journal of Learning Disabilities, 33*(3), 239–256.

Kessler, R. C., Duncan, G. J., Gennetian, L. A., Katz, L. F., Kling, J. R., Sampson, N. A., . . . Ludwig, J. (2014). Associations of housing mobility interventions for children in high-poverty neighborhoods with subsequent mental disorders during adolescence. *JAMA, 311*(9), 937–948.

LaPrairie, J. L., Schechter, J. C., Robinson, B. A., & Brennan, P. A. (2011). Perinatal risk factors in the development of aggression and violence. *Advances in Genetics, 75*, 215–253.

Lee, R., & Coccaro, E. (2001). The neuropsychopharmacology of criminality and aggression. *Canadian Journal of Psychiatry, 46*(1), 35–44.

Leve, L. D., & Cicchetti, D. (2016). Longitudinal transactional models of development and psychopathology. *Developmental Psychopathology, 28*(3), 621–622. doi:10.1017/s0954579416000201

Lozier, L. M., Cardinale, E. M., VanMeter, J. W., & Marsh, A. A. (2014). Mediation of the relationship between callous-unemotional traits and proactive aggression by amygdala response to fear among children with conduct problems. *JAMA Psychiatry, 71*(6), 627–636.

Marsh, A. A., Finger, E. C., Mitchell, D. G., Reid, M. E., Sims, C., Kosson, D. S., . . . Blair, R. (2008). Reduced amygdala response to fearful expressions in children and adolescents with callous-unemotional traits and disruptive behavior disorders. *The American Journal of Psychiatry, 165*(6), 712–720.

Media violence. (2009). *Pediatrics. 124*(5), 1495–1503. doi:10.1542/peds.2009-2146

Merriam-Webster. (2006). *Merriam-Webster's dictionary of law.* Springfield, MA: Author.

Meyer-Lindenberg, A., Buckholtz, J. W., Kolachana, B., Hariri, A. R., Pezawas, L., Blasi, G., . . . Callicott, J. H. (2006). Neural mechanisms of genetic risk for impulsivity and violence in humans. *Proceedings of the National Academy of Sciences, 103*(16), 6269–6274.

Müller, J. L., Sommer, M., Wagner, V., Lange, K., Taschler, H., Röder, C. H., . . . Hajak, G. (2003). Abnormalities in emotion processing within cortical and subcortical regions in criminal psychopaths: Evidence from a functional magnetic resonance imaging study using pictures with emotional content. *Biological Psychiatry, 54*(2), 152–162.

Panksepp, J. (1998). *Affective neuroscience: The foundations of human and animal emotions.* Oxford: Oxford University Press.

Passingham, R. E., & Toni, I. (2001). Contrasting the dorsal and ventral visual systems: Guidance of movement versus decision making. *NeuroImage, 14*(1), S125–S131.

Plattner, B., Karnik, N., Jo, B., Hall, R. E., Schallauer, A., Carrion, V., . . . Steiner, H. (2007). State and trait emotions in delinquent adolescents. *Child Psychiatry & Human Development, 38*(2), 155–169.

Pliszka, S. R., Rogeness, G. A., Renner, P., Sherman, J., & Broussard, T. (1988). Plasma neurochemistry in juvenile offenders. *Journal of the American Academy of Child & Adolescent Psychiatry, 27*(5), 588–594.

Popma, A., & Raine, A. (2006). Will future forensic assessment be neurobiologic? *Child and Adolescent Psychiatric Clinics of North America, 15*(2), 429–444.

Poremba, C. (1975). Learning disabilities, youth and delinquency: Programs for intervention. In H. Myklebust (Ed.), *Progress in learning disabilities* (Vol. 3). New York: Grune & Stratton.

Prot, S., Gentile, D. A., Anderson, C. A., Suzuki, K., Swing, E., Lim, K. M., . . . Liuqing, W. (2014). Long-term relations among prosocial-media use, empathy, and prosocial behavior. *Psychological Science, 25*(2), 358–368.

Quinn, M., Rutherford, R., Leone, P., Osher, D., & Poirier, J. (2005). Youth with disabilities in juvenile corrections: A national survey. *Exceptional Children, 71*(3), 339–345.

Raine, A. (2013). *The psychopathology of crime: Criminal behavior as a clinical disorder.* London: Elsevier.

Raschle, N. M., Menks, W. M., Fehlbaum, L. V., Tshomba, E., & Stadler, C. (2015). Structural and functional alterations in right dorsomedial prefrontal and left insular cortex co-localize in adolescents with aggressive behaviour: An ALE meta-analysis. *PloS One, 10*(9), e0136553.

Saxena, K., Howe, M., Simeonova, D., Steiner, H., & Chang, K. (2006). Divalproex sodium reduces overall aggression in youth at high risk for bipolar disorder. *Journal of Child & Adolescent Psychopharmacology, 16*(3), 252–259.

Slagt, M., Dubas, J. S., Deković, M., & van Aken, M. A. (2016). Differences in sensitivity to parenting depending on child temperament: A meta-analysis. *Psychological Bulletin, 142*(10), 1068–1110.

Stadler, C., Kroeger, A., Weyers, P., Grasmann, D., Horschinek, M., Freitag, C., & Clement, H.-W. (2011). Cortisol reactivity in boys with attention-deficit/hyperactivity disorder and disruptive behavior problems: The impact of callous unemotional traits. *Psychiatry Research, 187*(1), 204–209.

Stedman, T. L. (2006). *Stedman's medical dictionary.* Baltimore: Lippincott Williams & Wilkins.

Steiner, H. (2004). *Handbook of mental health interventions in children and adolescents: an integrated developmental approach.* San Francisco: Jossey-Bass.

Steiner, H. (2011). *Handbook of developmental psychiatry.* London: World Scientific.

Steiner, H., Carrion, V., Plattner, B., & Koopman, C. (2003). Dissociative symptoms in posttraumatic stress disorder: Diagnosis and treatment. *Child & Adolescent Psychiatry Clinics of North America, 12*(2), 231–249.

Steiner, H., Garcia, I. G., & Matthews, Z. (1997). Posttraumatic stress disorder in incarcerated juvenile delinquents. *Journal of the American Academy for Child & Adolescent Psychiatry,* 36(3), 357–365.

Steiner, H., & Hall, R. E. (2015). *Treating adolescents.* Hoboken, NJ: John Wiley.

Steiner, H., Medic, S., Plattner, B., Blair, J., & Haapanen, R. (October 2006). Predicting PIP and RADI aggression in incarcerated juvenile delinquents: Trama, affect and defensiveness. Paper presented at the annual meeting of the American Academy of Child and Adolescent Psychiatry. Honolulu, Hawaii. October 2006.

Sterzer, P., & Stadler, C. (2009). Neuroimaging of aggressive and violent behaviour in children and adolescents. *Frontiers in Behavioral Neuroscience,* 3, 35.

Sundheim, S. T., & Voeller, K. K. (2004). Psychiatric implications of language disorders and learning disabilities: Risks and management. *Journal of Child Neurology,* 19(10), 814–826.

Swann, A. C. (2003). Neuroreceptor mechanisms of aggression and its treatment. *Journal of Clinical Psychiatry,* 64(Suppl. 4), 26–35.

The damaging effect of media violence on young children. (2014, May). Session at the Pediatric Academic Societies annual meeting, Vancouver. https://www.aap.org/en-us/about-the-aap/aap-press-room/Pages/The-Damaging-Effect-of-Media-Violence-on-Young-Children.aspx

Ueno, K., & Schwenck, C. (2015). [Cognitive and affective perspective-taking in girls with conduct problems as a function of the callous-unemotional personality feature]. *Zeitschrift für Kinder-und Jugendpsychiatrie und Psychotherapie,* 43(5), 335–344.

Van Ryzin, M. J., & Leve, L. D. (2012). Affiliation with delinquent peers as a mediator of the effects of multidimensional treatment foster care for delinquent girls. *Journal of Consulting and Clinical Psychology,* 80(4), 588–596.

Veit, R., Flor, H., Erb, M., Hermann, C., Lotze, M., Grodd, W., & Birbaumer, N. (2002). Brain circuits involved in emotional learning in antisocial behavior and social phobia in humans. *Neuroscience Letters,* 328(3), 233–236.

Waldie, K., & Spreen, O. (1993). The relationship between learning disabilities and persisting delinquency. *Journal of Learning Disabilities,* 26(6), 417–423.

White, S. F., Marsh, A. A., Fowler, K. A., Schechter, J. C., Adalio, C., Pope, K., . . . Blair, R. J. R. (2012). Reduced amygdala response in youths with disruptive behavior disorders and psychopathic traits: Decreased emotional response versus increased top-down attention to nonemotional features. *The American Journal of Psychiatry,* 169(7), 750–758.

Suggested Reading and Resources

Cicchetti, D., & Cannon, T. (1999). Neurodevelopmental processes in the ontogenesis and epigenesis of psychopathology. *Development and Psychopathology,* 11, 375–393.

Development and Psychopathology. (1989–).

Kerig, P., Ludlow, A., & Wenar, C. (2012). *Developmental psychopathology,* 6th ed. Hoboken, NJ: John Wiley.

Oregon Social Learning Center. http://www.oslc.org/

Steiner H. (Ed.). (1996). *Treating adolescents.* San Francisco, Jossey-Bass.

Steiner, H. (Ed.). (2011). *The handbook of developmental psychiatry.* London: World Scientific.

Steiner H., with Rebecca Hall. (Eds.). (2015). *Treating adolescents,* 2nd ed. Hoboken, NJ: John Wiley.

5

Comprehensive and Integrated Treatment of Disruptive Behavior Disorders

5.1 Definitions

Treatment: "the medical management of a disease" (Stedman 2006). In the context of disruptive behavior disorders, it is prudent to add two qualifiers given the current state of knowledge in this field: comprehensive and integrated (Steiner, 2004). "Comprehensive" in this case means that we use all the appropriate tools we have at our disposal, be they biological, psychological, or social. "Integrated" refers to the fact that all of these parts of our therapeutics are combined to form a rational whole, not a thoughtless accumulation of interventions. One reason that understanding the meaning of such terms is important in the case of disruptive behavior disorders is due to the fact that we are facing truly biopsychosocial disorders that emerge through a multiplicity of causal loops. Any of these loops need to be disrupted in order to bring about progress and healing. We hinted at this state of affairs when we discussed our current nomenclature in chapter 2 and the various etiologies thought to be involved in the pathogenesis of disruptive behavior disorders (DBDs).

Comprehensive, integrated treatment: the rational consequence of our current knowledge, especially in those children and adolescents with a persisting and severe symptomatology. When it comes to disruptive behavior disorders, the whole is greater than the sum of its parts; thus relying on premature orthodoxy and reductionism is ill advised when we are treating these patients. Unfortunately, psychiatry has no penicillin to offer to eradicate bacteria that underlie DBDs. While this makes our job as physicians and therapists more complicated, there is no reason for therapeutic nihilism. Presently, we do not have a knowledge base that allows us to easily eradicate these disorders, due in large part to the fact that necessary studies are complex in design and difficult to carry out. That said, we are in a much better position now, in 2017, than we were 20 years ago when most treatment studies were located in the criminological literature and carried out by nonphysicians. A growing body of research has contributed greatly to our understanding of the diagnosis, etiology, and new therapeutics. Fortunately, the impact of this research is increasingly felt, as the discussion of the current treatment outcome literature of DBD in this chapter will show.

Randomized double blind placebo controlled clinical trials : often referred to as "the gold standard" of evidence-based medicine. In recent years, the literature has placed an increased emphasis and reliance on such trials. These studies are often thought of as the *sine qua non* to establish any particular intervention as efficacious and effective, a very laudable goal. Most treatments in medicine do not reach such a lofty standard unless there have been many investigations over many years, even decades. For complex reasons we discussed in chapter 1, in the past 50 years there have been many obstacles to the study of antisocial behavior and its disorders. Despite such past obstacles, there is now a rapidly building body of knowledge we can refer to as we make treatment decisions to help these youngsters and their families. This body of knowledge has a reasonable degree of support, showing some promise to lead to positive outcomes.

In the past decade it has also become clear that randomized double blind placebo controlled clinical trials have their own set of limitations, which we discuss in some detail in our handbook of mental health interventions (Steiner, 2004). Just to mention a few, they usually have stringent exclusion/inclusion criteria, which very often result in a rather "purified" cohort being studied, which does not always map onto the patient profiles seen in private practice or clinics. Relying on such exclusive cohorts very often leads to overly optimistic outcomes because of the more limited complexity of the cases studied.

Naturalistic studies: a time-honored stream of information in medicine that complements randomized double blind placebo controlled clinical trials, especially helpful when the latter are prospective (i.e., studies where researchers follow patients for some period of time after the study has completed) of large cohorts in clinics and practices. Others include *case series* (i.e., a collection of clinical cases that have been evaluated and treated in a similar fashion) examining promising interventions, and *case studies* (i.e., reports on carefully studied and treated individual patients), which can highlight the complexities encountered by the clinician and complement the clinician's practice-based evidence to round out the picture.

Consensus reports and *practice parameters*: important and weighty sources of information for clinicians. An example is our work as the Stanford-Howard-American Academy of Child and Adolescent Psychiatry (AACAP) work group

(Connor et al., 2006; Jensen et al., 2007). Such efforts involve large numbers of researchers, teachers, and clinicians who reach consensus as to what constitutes best practice. These reports are informed by empirical studies and clinical experience, generating concrete steps and clinical algorithms to help us move forward when empirical evidence is lacking.

In our review of the field, we draw on all of the sources of information described here. We rely on the two consensus reports referenced earlier in particular as we discuss the clinical implications and some of the controversies within the field relating to DBDs. We are fortunate to have two recent and rigorous reviews from Canada, which resulted in a practice parameter (Gorman et al., 2015; Pringsheim, Hirsch, Gardner, & Gorman, 2015a, 2015b). We also refer to the National Institute for Health and Care Excellence (NICE) Guidelines for Conduct Disorder published 2013 and—to some extent—refer to recommendations from existing European guidelines for conduct disorder (Association of the Scientific Medical Societies Germany). Prior to reviewing and summarizing the available evidence on all forms of treatment of DBDs, definitions and descriptions of the most relevant psychosocial treatment approaches are presented.

To begin, more knowledge is needed on whether positively evaluated intervention approaches are also efficient in real-world settings and what can be recommended to practitioners when even the best of available evidence-based programs do not work. Furthermore, there is increasing interest in the effectiveness of interventions provided to adolescents with serious behavior and emotional problems, including law violations within residential care, as such adolescents are often transferred to these specialized institutions. **Residential care** is an umbrella term, capturing various forms of residentially based living arrangements, from small group homes to large institutions, across three service systems: child welfare, mental health, and juvenile justice.

Most of the existing, carefully evaluated interventions for CD/oppositional defiant disorder (ODD) are based on behavioral or cognitive behavioral programs. Treatments using psychodynamic, psychoanalytic, or humanistic approaches have not been well evaluated and available evidence is suggestive. Cognitive behavior therapy (CBT) comprises a variety of methods aiming to help parents, children, and young people to understand links between their own behavior and its antecedents and consequences. CBT also prioritizes helping patients learn to identify the connections between their thoughts, feelings, and behaviors. Patients are taught to identify irrational and distorted thinking patterns and construct more adaptive belief systems. Cognitive behavioral approaches typically involve psychoeducation, teaching, and practicing self-management strategies and new skills. Thus CBT aims to enhance the patients' self-efficacy for achieving their own goals.

Various treatment approaches are differentially effective at different developmental stages. Furthermore, their effects seem to critically depend on the involvement of the family and social context in which they are applied. We must also be aware that there are often high barriers for affected children, adolescents, and families to receiving the treatment they urgently need. For example, severely affected children and adolescents are frequently referred to residential institutions, or even sent to correctional institutions, because of elevated risk of psychosocial maladjustment. Access to adequate, evidence-based, economical care and treatment is rare within these settings despite it being well known that children and adolescents who are under the care of the state show a higher rate of mental problems than their noninstitutionalised counterparts.

In addition, research also indicates that youths with disruptive behavior disorders represent a population with a high incidence of trauma-related symptoms due to early experiences of maltreatment and neglect. This fact has to be considered when delineating intervention plans. *Trauma sensitive care* includes the central idea that dysfunctional behavior can emerge as a result of an individual's adjustment to adverse, highly stressful life circumstances. In this sense, many kinds of currently problematic behaviors may be understood as initially adaptive coping strategies in response to negative situations. Thus comprehensive approaches should integrate aspects of trauma sensitive care, especially in residential care settings where staff workers are confronted with these adolescents showing severe behavioral and emotional dysregulation.

Family-based approaches, most importantly parent management training (PMT), child-focused approaches, such as problem-solving skills training, as well as multisystemic therapy and multidimensional family therapy are the most promising approaches in the treatment of CD and ODD.

Preventive intervention: a special set of interventions that deserve definition and discussion. The goal here is to intervene as effectively as possible before symptoms cluster into syndromes, or even before that, when we know that certain risk factors are present that could tip the balance into the direction of mental disorders if not eliminated. As we discuss, there are several interventions in this class that have empirical support in the treatment of DBDs.

Within this grouping, it is important to distinguish several levels of interventions.

Primary prevention (universal prevention): programs delivered universally and do not target a specific group that define its members as being at high risk within the population for developing the disorder.

Secondary prevention (selective prevention): selective prevention interventions aimed at individuals who are at high risk of developing the disorder or are showing very early signs or symptoms. Interventions tend to focus on reducing risk and strengthening resilience. Poverty, parental mental health problems, chronic familial conflict, early neglect or maltreatment, but also individual risk factors in the child, such as attention deficit hyperactivity disorder (ADHD) or temperament, are among the most important factors exposing children to risk for developing disruptive behavior disorders.

Tertiary prevention (indicated prevention): interventions aimed at those groups in which the given symptoms of a disorder are already evident but the full disorder has not yet developed. It is often difficult to distinguish between selective and indicated prevention. Parent training, for example, can be part of both selective and indicated interventions for prevention of conduct problems.

5.2 Review of Evidence—The Status of the Field

We will now provide a concise summary of the literature on treatment approaches for disruptive behavior disorders.

5.2.1 PREVENTION

Preventative interventions have long been a promising avenue for reducing maladaptive aggression in at-risk youth outside the clinical setting, for example, in the school setting. (Connor et al., 2006) A 2008 study by Webster-Stratton, Jamila Reid, and Stoolmiller looked at the impact of a program promoting school readiness among socioeconomically disadvantaged preschoolers and first-graders. Teachers were trained to use the Incredible Years Child Training curriculum (aka Dinosaur School). Incredible Years is an early intervention program originally developed as a clinic based treatment for youth with ODD and/or early onset conduct problems between the ages of three and seven. A modified curriculum, "Dinosaur School," was created for 153 teachers to implement in the classroom with over 1,700 students as a means of preventing conduct problems and increasing the school readiness of at risk youth. Overall, the children whose teachers participated in the intervention benefitted as evidenced by reduced behavior problems, better social skills, and more emotional self-regulation. This study and others like it show how early intervention can positively influence children's developmental trajectories (Webster-Stratton et al., 2008).

A 2012 meta-analysis (Candelaria, Fedewa, & Ahn, 2012) pooled over 30 years of data from 60 published and unpublished studies looking at the impact school-based anger management and related programs have on the negative outcomes associated with acts of aggression and other problem behaviors. The meta-analysis concluded that anger management and other programs designed to help address difficulties with impulse control provide modest benefits by reducing unfavorable social and educational outcomes for youth. Although the approaches utilized by the studies in this meta-analysis varied quite a bit, the ones that relied heavily on problem-solving strategies associated with CBT were particularly effective. This meta-analysis shows that common-sense approaches to helping children recognize and address maladaptive aggressive impulses (e.g., teaching problem-solving skills and emotional awareness) in a school setting have a notable positive impact on their functioning.

There is evidence suggesting that primary care providers, not just mental health clinicians, can play an important role in reducing teen aggression and substance abuse. For example, Cunningham and colleagues (2012) assessed the impact of a brief intervention that was previously shown to reduce alcohol use and violence among teens who presented to an emergency room for care due to medical illness or injury at six-month follow-up. In the original study, which looked at the interventions impact six months out, teens who were treated in a Flint, Michigan, emergency room were randomized to receive a computerized behavioral intervention, a live therapist–assisted computerized behavioral intervention, or nothing at all. The original study found that both the computerized behavioral intervention and the therapist-assisted version were effective in reducing incidents of violence and alcohol use based on participants' self-report. When Cunningham and colleagues (2012) extended the time to follow-up to 12 months, the therapist-assisted computerized intervention showed marked reductions in aggression and peer victimization; however, the effects on alcohol use and related behaviors had dissipated. Given that emergency rooms and primary care physicians are frequently the first point of contact for youth with mental health needs, the integration of mental health screening and ready access to mental health care in primary care settings is an important and rapidly evolving area of medicine.

When discussing programs aimed at preventing behavior problems, we must specifically focus on secondary intervention programs that seek to reduce those early risk factors that often confront socioeconomically disadvantaged families. In the late 1970s, David Olds began a nurse home visit program for new, and soon to be new, mothers from low-income backgrounds. This program was developed to help young mothers take better care of themselves and their babies. Over the past 30+ years, Dr. Olds's nurse home visit model has shown marked reductions in childhood injuries, maternal cigarette smoking during pregnancy, reduced incidence of child abuse, and increased workforce involvement among participating mothers (Goodman, 2006). A recent study published in the *Journal of the American Academy of Child & Adolescent Psychiatry* (Enoch et al, 2016) looked at the genetic and environmental factors that influenced the externalizing behaviors among a cohort of children born to first-time mothers from birth through age 18. In this study, the children whose mothers had received nurse home visits and were also rated higher in "self-efficacy" were better behaved at age two. Poorer maternal mental health and smoking were associated with externalizing problems (Enoch et al., 2016). Approaches to prevention like nurse home visits are a cost-effective and practical means of helping children avoid behavior problems in early childhood and maintain a healthy developmental trajectory.

One of the best-known preventive comprehensive programs is the Fast Track project, which comprises PMT with home visits but also child social-cognitive skills training, peer coaching and mentoring, academic skills tutoring, and a classroom social-emotional curricula. The program's impact was tested in a randomized controlled trial (RCT) that included 891 youth who screened positive at age five as being early starters in conduct problems. The children in this study were randomly assigned by school cluster to a 10-year intervention or control group.

The most important conclusion from this study is that a comprehensive, multicomponent developmental science–based intervention targeted toward early-starting conduct-problem children can significantly reduce adult psychopathology and violent crime. For instance, 19 years after identification and 8 years after the intervention ended, relative to control subjects, individuals randomly assigned to intervention displayed lower prevalence of externalizing problems, internalizing problems, and substance use problems; fewer violent and drug crime convictions; less risky sexual behavior; higher levels of well-being; and less frequency in spanking their children (Dodge et al., 2015). These data support the notion that selective preventive approaches starting early in childhood should be implemented broadly. The well-known Perry Preschool study was conducted from 1962 to 1967 with 123 preschoolers ages three to four years from disadvantaged backgrounds. The preschoolers were randomly divided into a group that received a high-quality preschool program and a comparison group who received no special preschool program. The study found that 40-year-old subjects who participated in the preschool program had higher earnings, were more likely to hold a job, were more likely to have graduated from high school, and, most interestingly, had committed fewer crimes than adults who did not have the preschool program. Also noteworthy, those who received the preschool program were 46% less likely to have served time in jail or prison and had a 33% lower arrest rate for violent crimes.

5.2.2 BIOLOGICAL AND PHARMACOLOGICAL TREATMENTS

Turning to a discussion of available biological and psychopharmacological interventions, we have to immediately acknowledge that this is the treatment of DBDs that has the weakest empirical data sets behind it. In principle, there should be many agents of specific interest, but, as a recent practice parameter from Canada concludes (Gorman et al., 2015), medications are second-line treatment of DBDs at best. This of course does not mean that these agents could not be better studied and more stringently evaluated; however, these studies are lacking. Most likely this is driven by the weakness of the diagnostic categories in this DBD grouping and the fact that, to this date, there still are only very limited indications given by, for instance the US Food and Drug Administration, despite some efforts of researchers, clinicians, and the interested public to change that (Jensen et al., 2007).

As of now, there are no current medications that are specifically indicated for the treatment of any of the DBDs, especially ODD or CD (Grant & Leppink, 2015). This is most likely a major obstacle in the further development and refinement of our data bases addressing biological treatments of antisocial behavior and aggression and the syndromes related to them, as grouped in the DBDs.

Unsurprisingly, these problems are reflected in the literature and the available guidelines for practice issued by professional bodies. When one of us (HS) wrote the AACAP practice parameter for the treatment of CD in 1997, we reported a paucity of properly designed and executed medication trials in this population, relegating medications to tools for managing crises and emergencies and to a supportive role of other carefully designed psychosocial treatment packages. The best case for medication use was in the context of another primary diagnosis (i.e., ADHD), where both overt (bigger effects) and covert aggression (overlapping with our current reactive/affective/defensive/impulsive [RADI] and proactive/instrumental/planned [PIP] constructs) could be demonstrated. The practice parameter called for a greater concerted effort to improve diagnostic criteria and the strong consideration of subtypification to improve this state of affairs. A review of available agents in 2004 showed only moderate progress in this regard (Ruths & Steiner, 2004). In 2007, one of us once again reviewed the field and recommended (in a practice parameter for the AACAP, this time addressing ODD) that medications were to be considered adjunctive, palliative, and noncurative, at best (Steiner & Remsing, 2007). There was some support for the use of antipsychotics, mood stabilizers, stimulants, and atomoxetine (the only newcomer to this line-up), especially when used—again—in the context of ADHD. From a practical point of view, antipsychotics were the most prescribed medications but often without sufficient rationale or empirical support.

Addressing the problem of psychopharmacological treatment from the broader perspective of juvenile aggression, the Stanford-Howard-AACAP task force was able to report more progress in the field (Connor et al., 2006). After reviewing the results of 154 randomized, controlled psychosocial treatment trials, 20 controlled psychopharmacology studies, 4 open-label medication studies, and 2 psychopharmacology meta-analyses, the task force arrived at very similar conclusions, as had another review in 2006 (Pappadopulos et al., 2006).

There was some support for the same list of agents as previously mentioned: atypical antipsychotics, mood stabilizers (lithium; divalproex), and stimulants and atomoxetine in the context of ADHD—again, with the latter delivering the best outcomes and greatest effect sizes. There were no new agents tested in the most rigorous fashion. The empirical data basis had widened considerably. Particularly welcome were the advent of two meta-analyses. Both reports, once again, suggested that medication trials should test the different phenotypes of aggression (cold vs. hot; PIP vs. RADI) as primary and secondary treatment outcome variables in specially designed trials, which up to that date were still lacking.

This persistent problem inspired our group at Stanford to re-examine the results of a previous randomized blind high-dose/low-dose comparison of the efficacy of divalproex sodium in severely males with CD with this particular subtypification in mind (Steiner, Petersen, Saxena, Ford, & Matthews, 2003).

As a first step, we reanalyzed the existing dataset by examining the impact of the mood stabilizer on key variables, which stood in direct relationship to PIP and RADI forms of aggression. We were able to show that negative emotional activation and self-regulation were significantly influenced by the medication in a positive direction: negative emotional activation was reduced, while ability to self-regulate was improved. Both the variables are in a strong relationship to RADI but not PIP aggression. As one of the study participants related: "Whenever they told me to count to 10 before I hit someone, I would get to three at best. With the medicine, I now get to nine. Then I still hit him, but not as hard." This is an excellent description of the type of drug effect we can hope for: this young man developed a longer fuse for his anger-fueled aggression but not necessarily a new strategy to deal with the situation. This would have to be imparted through other forms of treatment, based on cognitive-behavioral principles.

A second reanalysis of the data produced significant predictors of response to divalproex sodium in line with the findings of this first reanalysis: high negative emotional activation and low self-regulation, among other variables, at baseline predicted better response to divalproex sodium (Saxena, Silverman, Chang, Khanzode, & Steiner, 2005).

A third, more ambitious reanalysis confirmed these positive findings (Padhy et al., 2011). In this study, we divided the existing subject pool who all fulfilled Structured Interview criteria for CD into two subtypes—high distress and low distress—on the basis of their negative activation scores on a standardized instrument. The validity of this subdivision was further confirmed by the previous crime types committed by the subjects: high distress CDs were much more likely to be convicted of explosive, emotionally laden aggressive acts (e.g., manslaughter instead of first-degree murder). The new division produced a series of much-improved results, when compared to our original findings in the original study (Steiner et al., 2003). High distress CDs were significantly more likely to show improved outcomes after an average of eight weeks of treatment with divalproex sodium at therapeutic levels, as measured by the primary outcome measure, the clinical global improvement ratings by a blind clinician. Low-dose divalproex sodium produced a much smaller response. Low distress CDs did not respond to either low-dose or high-dose conditions. Furthermore, there were significant differences in outcome in the constituent variables for RADI aggression: negative activation and self-regulation. When treated with therapeutic levels of medication, the high distress CD group improved in the expected direction: negative activation was reduced, while self- regulation increased. These findings are very much in line with our expectations and in support of conducting medication trials with a similar array of primary and secondary outcome measures. This series of reanalyses also consistently provided results of greater significance compared to the original study, which was carried out in the traditional format (i.e., recruitment by diagnoses, randomization and low- and high-dose treatment control without particular subtypification).

A series of Canadian studies (Gorman et al.; Grant et al.) in 2015 provides an excellent and rigorous assessment of the psychopharmacology of DBDs. Two separate reviews summarize the available evidence supporting the use of several psychoactive compounds in the treatment of disruptive behavior and its disorders, as well as disruptive behaviors in the context of ADHD. The reviews summarize the evidence for stimulants, alpha-2 agonists and atomoxetine in part 1, then discuss the use of mood stabilizers and atypicals in part 2. After a systematic review of the recent literature, the group rated the quality of evidence using a standardized approach (the Grading of Recommendations, Assessment, Development and Evaluation Method). Two other systematic reviews and 20 RCTs were reviewed in part 1; 11 RCTs of antipsychotics and 7 RCTs of lithium and anticonvulsants were reviewed for part 2.

The findings supported the notion that the use of stimulants is supported by high-quality evidence. They have a moderate to large effect on oppositional behavior, conduct problems, and aggression in youth with ADHD, with and without ODD or CD. The reverse is not necessarily true; that is, stimulants in the absence of ADHD are probably not helpful in CD and ODD. We would add that the use of stimulants in the absence of ADHD—or even in its presence—in a population that has strong inclinations to exhibit antisocial and even criminal behavior (such as, e.g., selling the very drugs that they are being prescribed or abusing and diverting them in other ways [one must not forget that stimulants have very high street value and are highly addictive]) should be done with extreme care and awareness of its dangers.

Ideally, we would have at our disposal less potentially dangerous drugs; however, the available evidence shows much less support for their efficacy in the treatment of ADHD and DBDs. To start, the group found only very low-quality evidence that clonidine has a small effect on oppositional behavior and conduct problems in youth with ADHD, with and without ODD or CD. Furthermore, there is moderate-quality evidence that guanfacine has a small to moderate effect on oppositional behavior in youth with ADHD, with and without ODD. The best chances for this grouping of drugs comes from studies of the selective norepinephrine reuptake inhibitor atomoxetine: high-quality evidence shows that atomoxetine has a small effect on oppositional behavior in youth with ADHD, with and without ODD or CD.

The second review studied the data supporting several candidates for psychopharmacological treatment of DBDs, which should be taken into serious account because of their lack of street value and addiction and or dependence potential. While each one of them presents their own profile of special risks to the patient's health because of their side effect profiles, they do—with proper management of these side effects—represent a group of medications that should be seriously considered as candidates for intervention when there is a high degree of chaos, instability, and criminality in the social environment of the patient in question. Risperidone is the agent best supported by moderate-quality evidence to result in moderate to large effect on conduct problems and aggression in youth, mostly in those with subaverage IQ and ODD, CD, or disruptive behavior disorder not otherwise specified, with and without ADHD. High-quality evidence supports its use in DBDs without intellectual disabilities resulting in moderately positive outcomes. All this has to be carefully weighed against the fact that this drug and similar ones have potentially very serious side effects on maturation and metabolic status. Again, we would recommend extreme vigilance and tight follow-up if this and similar medications are used, considering the accompanying lack of structure in the psychosocial environments of this population. However, the risk for diversion, abuse, and criminal activities associated with these drugs is much less than with stimulants.

The remainder of drugs in the second review is supported only by low-quality studies, referring to haloperidol, thioridazine, quetiapine, divalproex, and lithium in aggressive youth with ODD or CD. The low quality derives mostly from the lack of RCTs with a large subject pool and sufficient length of follow-up. Carbamazepine should be eliminated from consideration altogether, because it is indistinguishable from placebo in the one study that tested its efficacy. There is very-low-quality evidence that carbamazepine is no different from placebo for the management of aggression in youth with CD.

Following these comprehensive and rigorous reviews, the Canadian group constructed a practice parameter for DBDs that in essence agrees with the recommendations we have given so far for the medication treatment of DBDs. As previously mentioned, we still are in the position of classifying medications as second-line treatment of DBDs in cases where insufficient progress has been achieved with psychosocial and individual psychological treatments. In the context of ADHD, stimulants are strongly recommended. Other compounds, such as atomoxetine and alpha 2 agonists, are only conditionally recommended. Risperidone has the strongest support of the atypicals in the presence of ADHD should the patient tolerate stimulant treatment poorly. This support also extends to cases where there is no comorbid ADHD, but, as we have discussed, many caveats apply, because of the potentially grave side effects, which reduce the support to conditional. In our opinion, the use probably should be restricted to acute antisocial and aggressive behavior that engenders danger to others and self. The use also should be time limited. The use of either quetiapine, haloperidol, lithium, or carbamazepine is not recommended at all, given the poor empirical data backing up these medications and the severe side effects, especially in maturing patients.

Still, almost completely lacking are studies that examine the sequential use of different treatments or medication compounds—even in the considerably more mature literature of ADHD. There are some rare exceptions, which should be regarded as a window into the future of a more sophisticated psychopharmacology for children and adolescents (Steiner & Karnik, 2009).

An important study by Waschbusch, Carrey, Willoughby, King, and Andrade (2007) looked at the effects of combination treatment consisting of behavioral therapy with or without the addition of stimulant medication on children with conduct problems and ADHD, approximately half of whom were also classified as having callous–unemotional traits. They discovered that children with the triad of ADHD, conduct problems, and callous–unemotional traits responded poorly to behavioral therapy alone relative to the study participants who lacked callous–unemotional traits. However, the behavior of youth with ADHD, conduct problems, and callous–unemotional traits approximated that of the study participants who lacked callous–unemotional traits when stimulant medication was administered in conjunction with behavioral therapy. This study makes a compelling argument for including stimulant medication in the treatment plan for youth with ADHD, conduct problems, and callous–unemotional traits. It is worth mentioning that this study did not look specifically at stimulant medication's impact on the incidence of hot versus cold acts of aggression in youth with ADHD, conduct problems, and callous–unemotional traits. However, its results underscore the significant benefits stimulant medication can have on problem behaviors in youth with callous–unemotional traits, conduct problems, and ADHD (Waschbusch et al., 2007).

Similar recommendations also come from the NICE group in the UK. According to the NICE guideline, risperidone should be prescribed for CD and severe aggression with emotional dysregulation only for a short treatment phase in case no other psychosocial intervention was successful. The group issues similar caveats regarding side effects in the context of long-term treatment, stating that risks outweigh the benefits (weight gain, extrapyramidal side effects, tiredness, drowsiness, increase of prolactin level). In some cases, Alpha-2 agonists, such as guanfacine and clonidine, may be helpful in treating aggressive behaviors in the context of ADHD.

Additional studies report results in line with all these recommendations. A meta-analysis conducted by Schwartz and Corrlell (2014) included 25 controlled trials that investigated the efficacy of atomoxetine for treating children and adolescents with ADHD and symptoms of ODD. Results indicated atomoxetine treatment was superior to placebo for reducing overall ADHD symptoms and showed a medium effect size for reducing oppositional behaviors associated with ODD (Schwartz & Correll, 2014). Thus we, in accordance with the NICE guideline, recommend the use of methylphenidate or amphetamine salts for treating ADHD and comorbid ODD/CD. Nonstimulants (atomoxetine or guanfacine) could be a pharmacologic treatment options as well, although the evidence base for atomoxetine is stronger.

Gadow et al. (2014) compared treatment effects of parent training and stimulant medication plus a placebo with that of parent training, stimulant medication, and risperidone among youth who displayed behavior problems that included symptoms of ADHD, ODD and CD. Youth whose problem behaviors were targeted by treatment with risperidone in addition to stimulant medication and parent training displayed small to moderately greater effect sizes than those who did not receive risperidone (Gadow et al., 2014).

Grant and Leppink's (2015) recent review points out that 15 controlled studies have looked at medication treatments for youth with CD, many of whom had an accompanying diagnosis of ADHD. The mood stabilizer medication lithium has shown efficacy in seven studies of youth with CD. Haloperidol, an older antipsychotic medication, has also shown efficacy. However, Grant and Leppink point out that both medications have been associated with cognitive deficits that may have been side effects, and, as such, they should only be given as a last resort when other treatment options have failed. Divalproex has also shown some promise in treating youth with CD, although none of these studies had a placebo arm. Its side-effect profile, especially in young women, is also of concern.

Very little research has been conducted on medication treatments for intermittent explosive disorder. In fact, a recent review article stated that only five controlled studies have specifically focused on medication treatments for intermittent explosive disorder (Grant & Leppink, 2015). One large randomized double blind placebo controlled clinical trials involving 100 youth found that fluoxetine was helpful in reducing irritability and impulsive aggression. Another study has shown that the anticonvulsant medication oxcarbamazepine has some efficacy in reducing impulsive aggression associated with intermittent explosive disorder. Additional anticonvulsant medications, divalproex and levitracetam were not shown to curb aggressive behavior associated with intermittent explosive disorder in a significant way.

In the only medication trial designed specifically for kleptomania, oral naltrexone was found to reduce overall symptomatology in the 25 patients who participated as measured by the Yale-Brown Obsessive Compulsive Scale Modified for Kleptomania (Grant & Leppink, 2015). Naltrexone was well tolerated by the participants of this study. One open label trial of the selective serotonin reuptake inhibitor escitalopram was associated with lower relapse rates. Case reports are all we have to go on in regard to medication and psychological treatments for pyromania. The current literature does not suggest any specific recommendations.

Special mention should be made of a gradually building body of literature that examines the efficacy of biological treatments of antisocial and aggressive behavior in the context of other primary diagnoses. The Canadian reviews discussed specifically introduce this topic in regard to ADHD, which delivers the most robust responses. For youth who meet criteria for both ODD and ADHD, stimulant medications have been effective in addressing the symptoms of both conditions. This has been known at least since 2002. Connor et al. (2002) revealed in a meta-analysis that included 28 studies that the overall weighted mean effect size was 0.84 for overt and 0.69 for covert aggression related behaviors in ADHD (Connor, Glatt, Lopez, Jackson, & Melloni, 2002). Thus stimulant effects for aggression-related behaviors in ADHD have effect sizes akin to those for the core symptoms of ADHD. Similarly, the results of a meta-analysis conducted by Epstein, Fonnesbeck, Potter, Rizzone, and McPheeters (2015) showed modest to high effect sizes for stimulants in addressing oppositional behaviors and other symptoms associated with CD among children with ADHD, regardless of whether they met full criteria for CD diagnosis. Spencer and colleagues (2006) investigated the efficacy of amphetamine salts in children and adolescents ages 6 to 17 years with ODD, 79% of which had a comorbid ADHD. The treatment with amphetamine salts resulted in a significant reduction of oppositional defiant behavior. In addition, Klein and his group (1997) showed that methylphenidate was effective in the treatment of CD independent of comorbid ADHD or ADHD severity. One important additional recommendation regarding ADHD medication that applies to medication and psychotherapy in general, however, is that the phenotype of aggression has to be taken into consideration. While acts of cold aggression (PIP) tended not to respond as robustly to stimulant medications, there is evidence suggesting that a special case can be made for the use of stimulant medication in youth with callous–unemotional traits and ADHD (Spencer et al., 2006).

There are similar findings in other diagnoses, such as bipolar disorder, intellectual disabilities, and potentially trauma related psychopathology, such as posttraumatic stress disorder (Steiner et al., 2007). Substance use disorders, anxiety disorders, autism spectrum disorders, and schizophrenia all have been reported to be associated with maladpative aggression and antisocial behavior. As the treatment of each of these disorders becomes increasingly specific, it will be very interesting to see if the ADHD example applies: will these disruptive behaviors respond to targeted interventions, as they clearly do in ADHD? Our group has generated preliminary evidence that this most likely will be so in the case of bipolar disorder (Saxena, Chang, & Steiner, 2006; Saxena, Howe, Simeonova, Steiner, & Chang, 2006).

In sum, the domain of biological treatments for DBDs is showing some progress in the past 10 years; however, much more work is needed to arrive at more conclusive results that will guide the clinician in a more positive direction. Problems with the current taxonomy, which we discussed extensively in chapter 2, leave us with considerable uncertainty in this domain of treatment. Our diagnoses are too broad, heterogenous and of uncertain relationship to our biological understanding of antisocial and aggressive acts. Such uncertainty also has prevented the field from obtaining an indication, which in turn results in decreased monetary support for the necessary studies.

We have same reasonable theoretical leads as to which neurophysiological factors would be suitable targets (e.g., increase in serotonin and GABA to foster self-regulation and impulse control, reduction of excitatory neurotransmitters such as dopamine, just to name a few). There is a potential line-up of subtypes that could help us move beyond this stagnation in research—the callous–unemotional dimension and the hot/cold aggression subtypes, which most likely would lead us to more positive results. But in the meantime, we have to be content with the consensus in the field that biological interventions are supportive and second line, except in other primary diagnoses (ADHD) where disease-specific interventions (stimulants and nonstimulants) have been shown to produce positive results.

For now, the clinician is best advised to follow the various practice parameter suggestions as summarized. In addition, Pappadopoulos and colleagues (2003) have issued a reasonable way to proceed when faced with disruptive behavior and its syndromes. Figure 5.1 summarizes these recommendations.

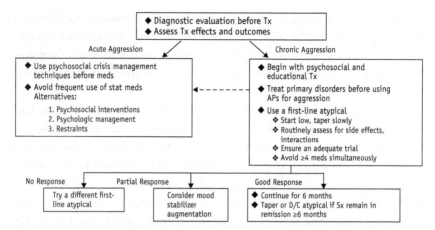

Figure 5.1 Consensus panel recommendation as to the best way to proceed with antipsychotic treatment of DBDs. Adapted from Pappadopulos et al. (2003).

5.2.3 PSYCHOLOGICAL INTERVENTIONS TARGETING THE INDIVIDUAL

Programs that intervene with individual children include those that seek to improve social skills and are often referred to as social skills training. Social skills training approaches set out to help children utilize social behaviors that foster and maintain positive responses from others.

Child-focused approaches are recommended for school-age children (NICE, 2013). Although some social skills training programs might be delivered individually, most of the existing programs have been evaluated in group settings. Such programs seek to improve social skills by focusing on the control of negative thoughts or moods, such as anger management training. Much of the available evidence indicates that these kind of interventions are most effective when therapists refer to real-life situations that are meaningful to youth and when techniques like role-play and practicing in vivo are utilized. The Anger Coping Program (Lochman et al., 2001), the Coping Power Program (Lochman & Wells, 2002; Lochman & Wells, 2003; Lochman & Wells, 2004), and the Problem-Solving Skills Program (Spivack, Platt, & Shure, 1976) are some of the best-known and best evaluated skills training programs. There is also a long history of problem-solving training programs that aim to enhance the social and emotional skills for entire classrooms of children.

Over the past decade there has been increased use of Dialectical Behavior Therapy (DBT) to target aggressive and self-destructive behaviors among youth. DBT was originally developed as an approach for treating patients with borderline personality disorder (Linehan, 1993). DBT is a treatment modality that aims to enhance emotion regulation strategies. DBT also relies heavily on a group therapy component. The aim of standard DBT modules is generally to teach and/or improve upon existing emotion regulation strategies, distress tolerance, and mindfulness. However, it is now increasingly applied to severe disruptive behavior, including in particular those living in correctional facilities (Berzins & Trestman, 2004; Quinn & Shera, 2009). For instance, some DBT modules have been modified specifically to target the the emotional insensitivity of patients diagnosed with DBDs and even antisocial personality disorder to promote positive emotional attachments and empathy toward others (McCann, Ball, & Ivanoff, 2000). An important aspect of the DBT modules described, in addition to the group skill training that patients receive, they also provide training and supervision for the professional team, including staff workers, who are regularly confronted with severely aggressive patients in their daily work. The in vivo coaching is implemented when a staff worker prompts a patient to use a DBT skill in everyday life. For example, a staff worker may prompt an adolescent who is quickly becoming more upset to use a breathing technique learned through DBT to cope with his negative emotions as a means of preventing an angry outburst. Furthermore, the generalizability of learned skills is attained though in vivo coaching, which is another important strategy in DBT.

The implementation of evidence-based skills training grounded in comprehensive training and supervision for staff is a promising means of avoiding staff burn out and/or turnover, thereby better ensuring continuous care for severely affected adolescents placed in correctional facilities as well as residential care settings. Addressing this important issue, NICE (2015) published a guideline on short-term management of aggressive behavior in mental health, health, and community settings (https://www.nice.org.uk/guidance/NG10). NICE's guideline clearly emphasizes the necessity of training staff in these settings to use de-escalation strategies (e.g., recognizing early signs of irritation or anger and knowing techniques for distraction, calming, and relaxation). Such de-escalation strategies can be applied to create safer environments for youth and staff in correctional facilities. Offering this kind of training and supervision to correctional staff workers is one way to help ensure that they are able to deal with challenging situations with a positive, respectful approach toward adolescents.

5.2.4 FAMILY-FOCUSED INTERVENTIONS

Family-focused interventions are part of the psychosocial interventions that still are the backbone of treatment of disruptive behavior across the entire developmental span from preschool to young adulthood. They comprise approaches that focus on the parents (PMT) or engage with the whole family, together with the child or young person (Functional Family Therapy [FFT], Brief Strategic

Family Therapy [BSFT]). Multidimensional family therapy additionally focuses on other community settings like school or peers. They are backed by some of the most solid evidence in the domain of treatment of DBDs and should definitely be considered as a group of first-line interventions when dealing with DBDs, especially if the patients are very young and or very dependent and threatened by their primary families. We discuss each in turn.

5.2.4.1 Parent Management Training

PMT comprises parenting interventions based on social learning theory to address parenting practices that have been identified in research as contributing to conduct problems. First, PMT aims to promote positive relationship between parents and children. Improving the parent–child relationship by using strategies based on social learning theory has become the cornerstone for the treatment of conduct problems in children. Helping parents learn the techniques of how to play in a constructive and warm-hearted way with their children helps them recognize their needs and respond sensitively. The children in turn begin to like and respect their parents more and become more secure in the relationship. Second, PMT aims to improve parenting skills. Parents are helped to reformulate difficult behavior in terms of the positive behavior they wish to see, so that they encourage wanted behavior rather than criticize unwanted behavior. For example, instead of shouting at the child not to cry, they would praise him whenever he tries to just say what he wants. Thus reinforcement of negative behavior is reduced, leading to the child engaging in more sociable behavior in response to praise and rewards. In addition, all available parenting programs help parents to establish clear-cut rules and simple commands. Emphasis is placed on teaching parents how they can effectively set boundaries and define consequences for unwanted behavior. Oftentimes parents do not feel self-sufficient when confronted with aggressive or oppositional behavior, leading to difficulties regulating their own negative feelings. Thus parents are trained in stress-regulation strategies and communication skills in order to better deal with challenging daily situations with their children. In addition, reorganizing the child's day to prevent trouble can be an effective tool to reduce stress and enhance a positive climate within the family. The Incredible Years, Triple P, and Parent–Child Interaction Therapy are some of the most effective PMT approaches.

PMT can be held in a variety of settings, including the hospital, clinic, community, or home. PMT can also be conducted either in groups, typically of 6 to 12 participants, or individually, as both formats seem to be equally effective; however, PMT in a group setting approach is more cost-effective. Some of the interventions, like Parent–Child Interaction Therapy, include the child, providing an opportunity to directly coach parents in challenging situations.

Garland, Hawley, Brookman-Frazee, and Hurlburt (2008) set about obtaining the opinions of experts on the common elements of evidence-based PMT. Their study found that experts reported that the most important PMT techniques included the use of rehearsal (e.g., parents rehearse new skills in session), the modeling PMT skills through live or imagined situations, and providing parents with homework or tasks to complete between sessions that are later reviewed with their therapist (Garland, et al., 2008).

5.2.4.2 Functional Family Therapy

FFT is an approach that was developed by James F. Alexander. Similar to PMT, FFT targets dysfunctional relationship patterns within a family. FFT aims include improving communication between parents and children, reducing interpersonal inconsistency, and increasing parents' levels of supervision and monitoring of their children. FFT also focuses on helping the family learn how to effectively negotiate house rules and the sanctions that are applied when said rules are broken.

In the first phase of FFT, dubbed the "engagement and motivation" phase, the therapist seeks to establish rapport with a family, foster a sense of hope, focus on interpersonal relations within the family instead of problem behaviors, and get the family to "buy in" to the approach. In the subsequent "behavior change" phase of FFT there is an emphasis on replacing rigid dysfunctional patterns of interaction among family members with a more flexible problem solving oriented style. In the final "generalization" phase of FFT the therapist helps the family apply what they have learned in a variety of contexts, explores how the family can respond to problems they anticipate arising in the future, and fosters links to local resources (e.g., school administrators, probation officers) that can lend the family support if needed (Henggeler & Sheidow, 2012).

5.2.4.3 Brief Strategic Family Therapy

BSFT is an approach based on Minuchin's structural and Haley's strategic family therapy models (Henggeler & Sheidow, 2012). BSFT's therapeutic focus is on the internal organization of a family including its level of cohesion and the roles played by different members. Conduct problems are viewed as resulting from the malfunctioning family system. In addition, this approach relies on the premise that all families, dysfunctional or not, seek to maintain their own equilibrium (i.e., the status quo). Any threats to this equilibrium, whether external or internal, tend to be met with resistance. In essence, BSFT seeks to help families find and maintain a new equilibrium or status quo. This approach was originally created in Miami, Florida, for use with youth with CD from Hispanic families. BSFT has since been studied among African American youth and youth with substance use disorders. The typical duration of treatment lasts around four months (Henggeler & Sheidow, 2012).

Evidence from several well-conducted meta-analyses confirms that behaviorally oriented PMT programs provide modest to moderate effects in reducing conduct problems among children in both the short term and the long term and across different informants, such as parents, professionals, and teachers (Bakker, Greven, Buitelaar, & Glennon, 2017; Devries et al., 2015; Menting et al., 2013; Sanders, Kirby, Tellegen, & Day, 2014). PMT in general is recommended to children ages 3 to 12 years (NICE, 2013). A recently published meta-analysis from Barlow et al. (2016) indicates that PMT might also be recommended in children younger than three years with externalizing behavior problems (Barlow, Smailagic, Ferriter, Bennett, & Jones, 2010).

Presently, there is no clear evidence indicating differences in PMT's effectiveness when the intervention is delivered in established service systems or under real-world practice conditions. Michelson et al (2013) conducted an meta-analysis analysis consisting of 28 RCTs that showed that an overall advantage for PMT compared with waitlist control conditions. No consistent relationships between specific real-world practice criteria (e.g., whether PMT was delivered in a service-oriented setting or a research setting or whether delivered by specialized therapists or nontherapists) and effect size estimates were found (Michelson, Davenport, Dretzke, Barlow, & Day, 2013). However, there was some indication for a greater effectiveness for PMT when delivered in established service delivery systems. In our opinion, manual guided evidence-based programs are a requirement for robust outcomes in routine clinical settings. The need to investigate the effectiveness of evidence-based interventions under real-world conditions also begs questions about what nonresponders or specific at-risk groups need in order to benefit from an intervention. Scott and Dadds (2009) have discussed some ideas from attachment theory, cognitive-attribution theory, and shared empowerment/motivational interviewing that could be helpful for enriching practitioners' ability to help families who are "stuck" during an intervention. Getting stuck in treatment seems to occur more often when specific risk factors are given (e.g., for children with high callous–unemotional traits; Scott & Dadds, 2009).

Somech and Elizur (2012) assessed the effectiveness of a co-parent training program in a RCT designed to provide early intervention to preschool-age youth deemed at risk for behavior problems. This program, called *Hitkashrut* (i.e., the Hebrew word for "attachment"), is a developmentally informed approach that seeks to capitalize on the powerful influence parents have on preschoolers and their developmental trajectories. The Hitkashrut approach was designed to specifically address callous–unemotional traits and "low effortful control" (i.e., difficulties inhibiting socially inappropriate behaviors) through parent training designed to foster enhanced attunement, responsiveness to their child's needs, and a more positive emotional tone. The strategies utilized in the Hitkashrut program included requiring that fathers be actively involved in co-parenting, emphasizing parental self-control in the face of situations that might normally trigger a volatile response, having parents provide healthy doses of positive reinforcement while maintaining consistent limits in response to inappropriate behaviors, and enhancing parent–teacher communication as a means of optimizing their child's behavior plan. These strategies were implemented, in part, by having parents increase the amount of quality time they spent with their child, encouraging parents to follow their child's interests and engage in more child-directed play, providing incentives for appropriate behaviors, and teaching parents skills to regain their composure before responding to their child's problem behaviors. The results of this study were quite encouraging. Families who received the intervention showed significant improvements, including reductions in callous–unemotional traits and increased effortful control, immediately following its completion. Additionally, the benefits persisted to a moderate degree on one-year follow-up. This study is important because it nicely illustrates the major impact that early intervention can have on children's developmental trajectories, even in youth especially prone to developing callous–unemotional traits (Somech & Elizur, 2012).

Thus, there is mounting evidence that children with callous–unemotional traits do show reductions in both these traits and their disruptive behavior, but typically they begin treatment with poorer premorbid functioning and can still end treatment with higher levels of antisocial behavior (Wilkinson, Waller, & Viding, 2015). A potentially essential factor leading to change in callous–unemotional traits and related antisocial behaviors over time for these children is parental warmth and involvement (Wilkinson et al., 2015; see Waller et al., 2013; Hyde et al., 2016). To have warm and sensitive parents might be the prerequisite to promote emotional learning and conscience development (Kochanska, 1997). Thus encouraging parents of children with callous–unemotional traits to build up positive relationships while helping them learn how to set limits seem crucial in breaking down the vicious circle of maladjustment.

The results for studies on other family-based interventions, such as FFT or BSFT are mixed but suggest promise in treating both status offenders and more serious juvenile offenders. A meta-analysis by Baldwin, Christian, Berkeljon, and Shadish (2012) compared family-based interventions like Brief Strategic Family Therapy (BSTF), Functional Family Therapy (FFT), Multidimensional Family Therapy (MDFT), and Multisystemic Therapy (MST) in the treatment of teen substance abuse and reduction of juvenile delinquency. All of these interventions were compared to a control group, some alternate form of therapy, or treatment as usual. This meta-analysis found that all four of the approaches showed modest effect sizes compared to treatment as usual or alternate approaches; however, effect sizes were modest. The effect of family therapy compared to control was larger but was not statistically significant. That said, this meta-analysis was underpowered (i.e., too small a sample size to detect meaningful differences between groups) and no conclusions could be drawn when comparing one of the four approaches versus the other or control groups (Baldwin et al., 2012).

5.2.5 SOCIOTHERAPEUTIC TREATMENTS

Multimodal (multisystemic, multidimensional) integrated and comprehensive approaches, such as Multisystemic Therapy (MST; Henggeler, Schoenwald, Borduin, Rowland, & Cunningham, 2009) and Multidimensional Treatment, Foster Care (MTFC; Chamberlain & Smith, 2005) are intensive family-based approaches that, unlike some of the other interventions we have discussed thus far, integrate community-based treatment aimed at impacting on the entire ecosystem or "milieu" in which young persons live (Chamberlain & Smith, 2005; Henggeler, Schoenwald, Borduin, Rowland, & Cunningham, 2009).

MST is a treatment model that was specifically developed for adolescents engaging in serious antisocial behaviors and their families. MST is based largely on social learning theory and uses a range of evidence-based interventions across home, school, and the local community environments. The aim of MST is to enable the "systems" around young persons to effectively manage them in a way that reduces antisocial behavior. A package of interventions is negotiated with the family and other key stakeholders that is complex, multifaceted, and time limited. A crucial aspect of MST is that despite its "packaged" nature, interventions are highly individualized to meet the needs of the young persons and their families. In order to provide this type of individualized care, MST comprises a 24-hour duty cover system provided by a multidisciplinary clinical team to ensure that families receive support from the therapist when crises are actually occurring. Major goals of MST include strengthening parental self-esteem and empowering them to take the reins within the family in a productive way. The great number of positive outcome studies on the efficacy of MST has led to the import of MST programs to more than 500 sites, including 10 nations in Europe.

MTFC uses an alternative means of providing an ecologically sensitive intervention for youth who display serious antisocial behaviors. MTFC intervenes by temporarily moving young people out of the families and into specifically trained foster families that are better equipped to address their needs. MTFC uses foster homes as the primary site of intervention. Similarly, foster families have access to resources and support services on a 24-hour basis, which are provided by a clinical team. Meanwhile, children's parents receive services as a means of bolstering their capacity to monitor and take care of their child in a safe and productive way on their return home.

A 2014 meta-analysis by van der Stouwe, Asscher, Stams, Deković, and van der Laan (2014) examined MST's effectiveness. MST was found to have note-worthy benefits in reducing juvenile delinquency and psychopathology, sub-stance use, and decreased out of home placements, among others. The results of this meta-analysis indicate that MST is more effective with youth under the age of 15; however, it may be effective for older teens when there is a greater empha-sis on addressing what is going on at school and a youth's peers. While offering some insights, this meta-analysis had limitations, which included the "inclu-sion of unpublished and nonrandomized studies" and "some studies of weak design" which "therefore had questionable validity "(van der Stouwe et al., 2014, p. 477). As one of the developers of MST, Dr. Scott Henggeler noted in a 2012 review article that therapists' adherence to MST protocols has been associated with better outcomes. For this reason, the organization that provides accredita-tion for MST programs, MST Services, monitors the fidelity of MST implemen-tation carefully (Henggeler, 2012).

A 21.9-year follow-up to a randomized clinical trial with serious and violent offenders found that the positive effects of MST reach as far as young adulthood. In this study, authors examined arrest, incarceration, and civil suit data in 176 serious and violent juvenile offenders who had been randomized to MST or individual therapy (IT) on average 20 years before (Sawyer & Borduin, 2011). Intent-to-treat analyses showed that felony recidivism rates were significantly lower for MST participants than for IT participants (34.8% vs. 54.8%, respec-tively) and that the frequency of misdemeanor offending was five times lower for MST participants. In addition, the odds of involvement in family-related civil suits during adulthood were twice as high for IT participants as for MST partici-pants. Further analyses revealed that the positive impact of MST can even extend to other members of the family (Wagner et al., 2014). This is of major interest as we can assume that psychosocial risk factors that are specifically addressed in MST (i.e., family dysfunction, negative communication, insufficient parental control) may also affect other family members and put them at risk for malad-justment as well.

Regarding the effectiveness of MDFT, one recently published randomized control trial conducted by Dakof and colleagues (2015) investigated the effec-tiveness of MDFT and group-based treatment. The group-based treatment in this study consisted of adolescent group skills training that incorporated motivational interviewing techniques. Both treatments, MST and the group-based treatment, were delivered by the juvenile drug court. During the inter-vention phase, youth in both treatments revealed high effects on reduction in delinquency, externalizing symptoms, rearrests, and substance use. During the

24-month follow-up, however, family therapy outperformed nonfamily based treatment in reducing criminal behavior and rearrests (Dakof et al., 2015). The results of Deković, Asscher, Manders, Prins, and van der Laan (2012) randomized control trial with 256 adolescents and their families who received either MST or treatment as usual are of interest. Deković et al. showed that MST enhanced growth in parental sense of competence and positive discipline and resulted in a decrease in adolescent externalizing problems. The results further supported a sequential pattern of change for positive discipline: Changes in parental sense of competence predicted changes in positive discipline, which in turn predicted decrease in adolescent externalizing problems.

Results of a recent meta-analysis indicate significant long-term effects of psychosocial intervention programs on youth antisocial behavior (Sawyer, Borduin, & Dopp, 2015). The reductions in antisocial behavior were evident for an average of four years following completion of interventions, with a handful of interventions demonstrating positive effects for more than a decade after they were delivered. Although results of this meta-analysis from 66 controlled prevention and therapy trials showed that participants demographic variables (i.e., age, gender, and ethnic background) did not moderate the size or direction of intervention effects on antisocial behavior, when considered separately some differential effects have been discovered. For example, peer group interventions were less effective when samples contained more boys or older youths than when samples had fewer boys or younger youths. This result is of major interest as there still is an ongoing debate whether peer group interventions might have an iatrogenic effect because of the risk of reinforcing each other's antisocial behavior. Although there is some indication that peer interventions might be more effective for children than for adolescents, we are more optimistic and in favor of conducting more controlled studies in this age group.

Although significant effects on youth antisocial behavior have been demonstrated under both experimental (i.e., efficacy) and practice (i.e., effectiveness) conditions, results from the meta-analyses conducted by Sawyer, Borduin and Dopp (2015) further indicate that effect sizes might be slightly higher when interventions are provided within established academic settings with intensive training and supervision compared to effectiveness trials conducted in community. Thus one major conclusion from this result is that when implementing interventions in real-world clinical and nonclinical settings, sufficient training and supervision should be guaranteed.

In line with Sawyer and colleagues (2015), we would like to raise another important issue for discussion. Contrary to the fact that there now is sufficient knowledge regarding evidence-based interventions, their dissemination still remains low in mental health, juvenile justice, and education service systems.

Still, interventions that have been found to have even null or even negative effects continue to be widely used (e.g., the Scared Straight program, which entails visits by at-risk youth to adult prisons, where youth hear about the harsh reality of prison life from inmates).

5.2.6 PSYCHOTHERAPY FOR OTHER DISORDERS MORE RECENTLY INCLUDED IN THE DBD CLUSTER

In contrast to the ODD and CD literature, there is a dearth of studies of psychosocial interventions in DBDs other than CD and ODD. There has only been one study that looks specifically at the efficacy of psychotherapy for youth with intermittent explosive disorder (Grant & Leppink, 2015). Unsurprisingly, this study found that CBT or group therapy was much more helpful than being a waitlisted member of the control group. The literature on psychological interventions for kleptomania consists of a handful of case reports involving convert sensitization and/or exposure and response prevention exercises. As stated previously, the only literature on treatments for pyromania are case reports.

5.2.7 DBD TREATMENT IN RESIDENTIAL CARE

As we mentioned earlier in this chapter, adolescents with severe DBDs are often placed in residential care. There are very few studies investigating the effectiveness of residential care or studies comparing residential care to well-evaluated community-based therapies such as MST or MTFC. Other concerns about benefits of residential care have been raised: the potential for abuse within institutions (Colton, Vanstone, & Walby, 2002), iatrogenic effects such as negative peer processes (Dishion, McCord, & Poulin, 1999), lack of professional training and high turnover rates, and the failure of residential care services to adequately involve the family (Colton, Vanstone, & Walby, 2002; Dishion et al., 1999).

Although the rate of juvenile offending in the United States has trended downward in recent years, the proportion of girls involved in the juvenile justice system has risen significantly over the past 30 years, including a 50% increase in juvenile arrests of girls, with girls accounting for 29% of all juvenile arrests (Maughan, Rowe, Messer, Goodman, & Meltzer, 2004; Puzzanchera, 2013).

Thus one important question to answer fairly soon is: Which evidence-based interventions have been implemented in residential care settings, how effective are they, and are there programs specifically tailored for girls? James and colleagues looked into this question in respective outcome studies, published from 1990 to 2012. Ten interventions matching a priori criteria were identified, among others: adolescent community reinforcement approach, aggression replacement training, dialectical behavioral therapy, ecologically based family therapy, eye movement and desensitization therapy, and FFT. Most of the interventions were behaviorally oriented or had a trauma focus. Outcomes were generally positive, establishing the relative effectiveness of these interventions with youth in residential care settings across a range of psychosocial outcome. However, there are some study limitations, including weak study designs and a lack of specificity about the elements of usual care. However, the meta-analyses conducted by de Swart et al. (2012) comprising 27 studies additionally demonstrates that providing youth in residential care settings with evidence-based treatment (CBT) is promising and might be as effective as community-based evidence-based therapy (MST, MDFT). There is some indication that, especially in girls, interventions involving the families might be more effective (Sawyer et al., 2015). Thus efforts to foster parental engagement also during residential care might be promising. However, barriers to parental engagement can be difficult to overcome, and treatments need to accommodate care without a parent component to ensure that all youth can receive the best treatments available regardless of their parents' ability or willingness to become involved in the treatment process.

There is a recognized need to transport evidence-based treatment to residential care settings and to overcome the variety of implementation barriers. Effective treatment of severely aggressive, rule-breaking, and unit-destructive behavior is crucial to the safe operation of the environment of the correctional facilities. This is of major relevance for staff workers dealing with adolescents who experience severe behavioral and emotional dysregulation and who often are not motivated for behavior change. The implementation of evidence-based intervention approaches within correctional or residential care facilities seems crucial both for a positive development of severely affected youth and for staff workers. Providing strategies for how to deal with challenging situations (e.g., oppositional behavior or resistance in adolescents) is essential in order to avoid staff burnout and high staff turnover and, as a negative consequence in adolescents, the risk of repeated experience of relationship break-offs.

Training staff to use motivational interviewing (MI) techniques might be helpful to qualify staff to deal with youth´s resistance and oppositional behavior. MI, originally developed by Rollnik and Miller (2012), aims to replace externally or coercive-driven communication strategies with a person-centered, collaborative guiding to elicit and strengthen motivation for change. MI may thus contribute to replace externally (or coercive) driven methods for motivating change that have been shown to elicit resistance with more effective strategies. A combination between MI and CBT seems particular promising because MI can develop offenders' motivation to change their maladaptive behaviors and

CBT provides the tools to effectively carry out this change. The fundamental principles and methodologies of MI have been applied and tested in various settings, and research findings have demonstrated its efficacy for a variety of diagnoses (Miller & Rollnick, 2012). MI has increasingly also been recommended for use by probation officers (Clark et al., 2006); offenders supervised with an MI approach have shown more significant positive changes in crime-related attitudes, as well as reduced endorsement of substance-related problems (Clark, Walters, Gingerich, & Meltzer, 2006; Harper & Hardy, 2000). In another study (Stein et al., 2006), incarcerated adolescents were randomly assigned to a brief (two-session) intervention of either MI or relaxation training. Postincarceration, those receiving MI had lower rates of drinking and of riding in a drinking driver's vehicle (Stein et al., 2006). In a quasi-experimental study, incarcerated offenders offered a brief MI intervention were compared to those receiving treatment as usual; at two-year follow-up, those in the MI condition showed significantly reduced rates of reconviction (57% vs. 78%; Anstiss, Polaschek, & Wilson, 2011).

NICE recently published a guideline on short-term management in mental health, health, and community settings that clearly strengthens the necessity of training staff in the use of de-escalation strategies (e.g., recognizing early signs of irritation or anger and knowing techniques for distraction, calming, and relaxation). In addition, de-escalation comprises goals to improve the physical environment of the correctional facility and to offer training and supervision for staff workers in order to ensure that they are able to appropriately deal with challenging situations and to maintain an encouraging positive, respectful approach toward adolescents.

5.3 Controversies and Future Steps

Existing findings support the use of psychological and family- and community-based psychosocial treatments for DBDs as first-line interventions. By comparison, the psychopharmacology of antisocial acts and aggression rests on much shakier evidence and has not matured further in the past decade. After a modest growth spurt between 1997 and 2007, there has been very little progress by any metric applied (Food and Drug Administration indications, new medications, stringent trials, application of biological or psychological subtyping to gain knowledge regarding types of medications chosen to be maximally effective, combination treatments, etc.). We are still in the position of just having tantalizing leads without a great deal of firm evidence. At best, some compounds are second-line treatments; at worst they are ineffective or even dangerous.

Most of this evidence refers to the treatment of CD and some to ODD specifically. However, there is a lack of literature comparing different types and combinations of intervention programs. A recent meta-analysis set out to examine which types of interventions for disruptive behavior disorders are most effective, those with a child only component, a parent only component, or multiple components. The interventions looked at in this meta-analysis included the Incredible Years–Parent Training, Parent Management Training Oregon Model, and MST, among others. All of the interventions with "multiple components" included in this meta-analysis included a parent component plus some combination of interventions involving the child, family, and/or school. Broadly speaking, interventions that involved parents alone or parents in conjunction with the child, family, and/or school had the greatest effect (Epstein et al., 2015). In our opinion, the results of this meta-analysis speak to the inherent complexity of DBD. For instance, if DBDs were a purely biologic or self-contained phenomenon, it would make sense if individual psychotherapy plus or minus medications would work equally well as interventions that rely on parental and school participation. What we know about these conditions is that individual therapy alone is rarely enough because it typically does not address the underlying family, neighborhood, academic, and other sociodemographic variables that contribute to the emergence and persistence of DBDs. In a larger review for the Agency for Healthcare Research and Quality, Epstein and colleagues (2015) additionally looked at data on pharmacologic interventions for DBDs. The final conclusion regarding medication was that antipsychotics and stimulant medications are effective in reducing CD and ODD symptoms over the short term; however, the phenotype of aggression has to be taken into account. In particular, we must consider how temperament may influence treatment response in DBDs (Stadler et al., 2008; Viding, Fontaine, & McCrory, 2012). Consistent with findings from other studies mentioned in this book, the behavior of children with callous–unemotional traits responded less robustly to discipline. In addition, the boys with callous–unemotional traits had reduced outward emotional expression in response to discipline as compared to children who lacked callous–unemotional traits. Children and adolescents with DBD and high callous-unemotional traits have also been known to be more refractory to intervention.

In 2005, Hawes and Dadds assessed the influence of a 10-week parent training course had on a group of four- to eight-year-old boys who met criteria for either ODD or CD. Children with callous–unemotional traits benefitted less from their parents' participation in the parent training course (Hawes & Dadds, 2005). A creative study by Stadler and colleagues (2008) looked at the issue of biology and disruptive behavior disorders from a unique angle; that is, whether a lower basal heart rate in youth with DBDs predicted poorer treatment response. Stadler and colleagues found that a lower basal heart rate predicted a significantly less favorable treatment response to a multimodal CBT program in youth with disruptive behavior disorders. While this study involved only 23 children with DBDs who were enrolled in an intensive day program that included parent training, the results complement a recent meta-analysis: Wilkinson et al. (2015) investigated in a meta-analysis the questions whether CU traits predict treatment success and whether interventions reduce levels of callous-unemotional traits. Although there was a mixed pattern of findings out of 15 control intervention trials, the evidence supports the idea that children with callous-unemotional traits do show reductions in both their callous-unemotional traits and conduct problems but typically begin treatment with poorer premorbid functioning and can still end with higher symptom levels.

If youth with callous–unemotional traits are less responsive to training interventions, what else can be done to maximize treatment effectiveness? As has been our mantra thus far, temperamental and personality traits, not mere diagnoses alone, have important implications for treatment selection and the likelihood of treatment success in DBDs. Probably more intensive and comprehensive interventions tailored to their unique emotional, cognitive, and motivational needs have to be developed for this specific subgroup. There is convincing evidence that PMT, particularly when delivered early in childhood, is capable of producing lasting improvement in callous-unemotional traits (Hawes, Price, & Dadds, 2014) (see also below p. 197 ff). Most important, parents should be continuously and consequently supported to work on a positive, warm parent–child relation as this is the prerequisite for emotional learning. This recommendation fits with the developmental biopsychosocial model we have espoused in this text. That is, the further upstream we are able to treat the difficulties of the children with DBDs, the greater the likelihood we will be able to get their developmental trajectory back on track.

In general, findings from recent meta-analysis (Epstein et al., 2015) clearly support that psychosocial interventions that include a parent component either alone or in combination with other components have the greatest probability of being most effective (Epstein et al., 2015). Based on the existing literature, we know that changes in child conduct problems are mediated by changes in parenting practices (reduced harsh and inconsistent parenting and improved positive parenting) and parent-reported stress, and this might be also especially true in children with both conduct problems and high callous-unemotional traits. In addition, we strongly encourage the development of new innovative intervention approaches that may be specifically tailored to the unique emotional, cognitive, and motivational needs of children with high callous unemotional traits aggression type.

Returning to our concern that we do not know much regarding the effectiveness of the combination of intervention programs (e.g. parent training +

child-based intervention versus child intervention alone), this is also true regarding the combination of psychosocial and pharmacological interventions. Up to now, there are no studies evaluating the efficacy of both behavioral and pharmacologic interventions compared to pharmacologic or behavioral interventions alone.

Due to symptom heterogeneity, the management of DBDs often entails a sequential, individualized approach whereby treatment (e.g., psychosocial, pharmacotherapy, or a combination) is adapted and readapted over time in response to the specific needs and evolving status of the individual. Given the fact that multipronged approaches are often used to treat DBD in clinical practice, studies investigating the combination of pharmacotherapy and psychosocial interventions are urgently needed. Clinicians who work with children with DBDs face an array of treatment approaches to combat a complex set of symptoms. In the coming years, it is incumbent upon our field to do a better job of developing precise guidelines to answer the important question: What treatments, and combinations thereof, work best for whom? A promising methodological approach to test the efficacy of an adaptive, sequential, or combined intervention is the use of a sequential multiple assignment randomized trial (SMART), which hopefully will be applied in future research studies more often (Almirall, Nahum-Shani, Sherwood, & Murphy, 2014).

Unfortunately, our field has not progressed very far over the past 10 years, making many of yesterday's recommendations today's most empirically supported interventions. In 2006 the Stanford-Howard-AACAP Workgroup on Juvenile Impulsivity and Aggression published a paper on the status of the field in regard to prevention, psychosocial, and pharmacologic interventions for youth prone to maladaptive forms of aggression in their two phenotypes, PIP and RADI. This suggestion has not reached the treatment outcome literature as of yet. Future studies on intervention effectiveness should also place more emphasis on considering aggression phenotypes. Such inquiries should include investigations of the moderating effects of cold and hot aggression and temperamental factors like callous–unemotional traits. Studies like this are needed in order to answer important questions about which treatments are most effective for certain subgroups.

We note that callous–unemotional traits do not necessarily bear a discernible relation to outcomes. This fact has to be taken into account not only for clinicians when delineating an intervention plan but also for the judicial system. Kolko and Pardini (2010), for example, studied outcomes associated with ADHD, callous–unemotional traits, and specific dimensions of ODD (e.g., hurtfulness, irritability) among 177 youth between the ages of 6 and 11. All participants met criteria for ODD or CD at intake and were enrolled in a modular treatment protocol or "treatment as usual." Unsurprisingly, the youth who met criteria for

CD at the outset were most likely have persistent symptoms of CD at posttreatment follow-up three years later. Interestingly, the youth who were labeled as having higher levels of ODD related "hurtfulness" (i.e., those who were rated as being frequently spiteful and vindictive) were more likely to develop treatment-resistant CD, juvenile delinquency (e.g., violence, theft, and/or vandalism), and other externalizing problems. Youth who happened to meet criteria for ADHD at the start of the study had an increased likelihood to develop ODD and had a tougher time socially. ODD-related irritability was associated with internalizing problems, higher degrees of overall functional impairment, and treatment-refractory ODD (Kolko & Pardini, 2010).

The most interesting finding from the Kolko and Pardini (2010) study, however, was that callous–unemotional traits did not bear any discernible relation to outcomes three years posttreatment. This finding was significant because it suggested that callous–unemotional traits might be fairly malleable over time, which, if true, has major treatment and legal implications. For instance, the US Supreme Court recently ruled in *Montgomery v. Louisiana* (2016) that sentencing an individual to life without the possibility of parole for crimes committed while under the age of 18 is unconstitutional, unless said individual is found to be "irreparably corrupt" or "permanently incorrigible." The *Montgomery* ruling expanded and made retroactive the US Supreme Court's decision in *Miller v. Alabama* (2012), which decreed that mandatory sentencing of juvenile offenders to life without the possibility of parole was unconstitutional. While a more recent meta-analysis showed that callous–unemotional traits are in fact associated with poorer treatment outcomes, the authors also concluded that certain parent training interventions can attenuate callous–unemotional traits, especially with early intervention (Hawes et al., 2014). These data indicating that callous–unemotional traits are not necessarily impervious to treatment are a source of hope for treatment providers and a call for forensic psychiatrists and psychologists to exercise great caution before suggesting that a juvenile offender is "irreparably corrupt" or "permanently incorrigible."

Finally, treatment studies should additionally investigate neurobiological correlates of treatment effects. This seems of major interest in order to better understand the underlying mechanism of treatment success on a neurobiological level. For example, Stadler and colleagues (2008) investigate the efficacy of a comprehensive skills training program for female adolescents with ODD and CD on emotion regulation both on a behavioral and a neurobiological level pre–post to intervention compared to treatment as usual (Kersten et al., 2016). Thus by integrating these research questions, we will be more and more able to define bottom-up (biology influences and changes in psychology and social causal loops) or top-down effects (psychology or social interventions have effects on biology).

5.5 Implications for Clinical Practice

As suggested by the sheer size of this chapter on treatment, previous statements regarding the treatment of antisocial, aggressive, and delinquent youths such as "nothing works" are not valid anymore (Lipton, Martinson, & Wilks, 1975). Existing findings from several meta-analysis support at least significant modest effects of psychosocial interventions on antisocial behavior. We are convinced that psychosocial interventions effectiveness could be increased if we aim to better tailor interventions to various aggression phenotypes. For instance, youth with callous–unemotional traits who have been shown emotionally and physiologically underreactive, particularly to others' distress, likely will not profit from the same intervention as youth with conduct problems and low callous–unemotional traits who are characterized by severe dysregulation and often were exposed to environmental risk factors, even maltreatment and neglect. Both subgroups need different intervention approaches.

We are also concerned about the fact that the proportion of youths who are given psychotropic medication to manage behavior problems has continued to increase over the past several decades, despite the fact that some of the most commonly used medications (e.g., antipsychotics) have a number of adverse side effects and only have moderate to modest support for their efficacy. Especially in residential care or forensic settings, the use of medication is common: Connor, Ozbayrak, Kusiak, Caponi, and Melloni (1997) showed that 75% of residential patients receive pharmacotherapy for aggression, 40% two or more medications.

Such idiosyncratic practices are not limited to biological interventions. The continued use of interventions that lack empirical support or have negative side effects, such as wilderness programs and Scared Straight, speaks to the considerable challenges associated with disseminating and implementing evidence-based psychosocial intervention programs for youth with DBDs. An increased implementation of evidence-based interventions needs effective strategies and strong cooperation between intervention developers, policymakers, and service systems.

Treating DBDs, we have to take into consideration the heterogeneity of the symptomatology ranging from impulsive and reactive forms of hot aggression to proactive and predatory forms of cold aggression. In addition, age of onset, comorbidity, and a multitude of psychosocial risk factors play a pivotal role for the final phenotype and course of these disorders. Thus, besides looking at individual temperamental factors that moderate treatment response, we also have to take into consideration the impact of familial risk factors like low socioeconomic status, family burden, parental mental health problems and parental stress. All of these factors are associated with a higher risk of negative parenting practices, child maltreatment, and even neglect. Thus we have to develop care plans with children and their parents in the context of any personal, social, occupational, housing, or educational needs. Given the complexity of risk factors described, comprehensive and integrated approaches within the family and community (e.g., school, peers) settings are recommended.

Treatment approaches that involve children's communities can even include visits to their kindergartens or elementary schools to provide therapeutic strategies and support teachers working with children displaying problematic behaviors. Community-based approaches can also involve bringing evidence-based approaches (e.g., problem-solving trainings) into the school setting. For instances in which the school is unable to effectively manage conduct problems despite additional support and adjunctive therapy for the child, clinicians can consider recommending that a child be moved to a unit specializing in the management of DBDs. The goal of such referrals should be to create an environment that is stable and predictable and improves the patient's self-esteem and relationships with prosocial peers. Repeatedly changing treatment providers and support service personnel should be avoided whenever possible.

We have to be aware that the treatment approaches described in this chapter are differentially effective at different developmental stages. Furthermore, the effects of interventions for DBDs depend heavily on the family and social context in which they are applied. Given the complexity of the disorder, there is no convincing evidence that unimodal child-focused approaches are likely to be effective in the treatment of severe or chronic DBDs. Interventions with a parent component, either alone or in combination with other components, including interventions in the community, are likely to have the largest effect. However, where parents are not coping or are actively damaging the child in an abusive relationship, it might be necessary to liaise with the social services department to arrange respite for the parents or a period of foster or residential care. It is important during this time to work with the family to increase their skills so that the child can return to the family. Where there is permanent breakdown, long-term fostering or institutional care might be necessary, but this should be the exception, not the rule.

Our knowledge regarding DBD treatment has expanded enormously within the past one to two decades. The evidence is convincing that programs based on the social learning theory such as PMT, MST, and MDFT, along with child-focused skills-training programs, are the best approaches in the treatment of DBDs. Nevertheless, there are still multiple implementation barriers when transporting these evidence-based intervention programs to the real-world setting.

Finally, it must be fairly acknowledged that there is a lack of evidence-based interventions in the transition from adolescence to adulthood, especially in high-risk patients. Data of the National Audit Office in England revealed that

80% of young people who leave residential care still face significant difficulties: More than 40% of 19-year-old care leavers are not in education, training, or employment, compared to 15% of their peers, and they often still have mental health problems. The majority of these young people would likely not seek help from mental health services or consult healthcare professionals. Thus innovative approaches should also consider e-mental health techniques as well as the use of social networks to better bring young people at risk to treatment and mental health services.

Still, over all we have many reasons to be optimistic. Looking at the rich toolbox at our disposal, we can say with some confidence "It is never too late and never too early" to help these most unfortunate youngsters and their families. And with continued interest, compassion, and constancy of purpose, we anticipate that a great deal of progress will be made in the next decade or two. We owe it to our patients and their families.

References

Almirall, D., Nahum-Shani, I., Sherwood, N. E., & Murphy, S. A. (2014). Introduction to SMART designs for the development of adaptive interventions: With application to weight loss research. *Translational Behavioral Medicine, 4*(3), 260–274.

Anstiss, B., Polaschek, D. L., & Wilson, M. (2011). A brief motivational interviewing intervention with prisoners: #when you lead a horse to water, can it drink for itself? *Psychology, Crime & Law, 17*(8), 689–710.

Bakker, M., Greven, C., Buitelaar, J., & Glennon, J. (2017). Practitioner review: Psychological treatments for children and adolescents with conduct disorder problems—a systematic review and meta-analysis. *Journal of Child Psychology and Psychiatry, 58*(1), 4–18.

Baldwin, S. A., Christian, S., Berkeljon, A., & Shadish, W. R. (2012). The effects of family therapies for adolescent delinquency and substance abuse: A meta-analysis. *Journal of Marital and Family Therapy, 38*(1), 281–304.

Barlow, J., Smailagic, N., Ferriter, M., Bennett, C., & Jones, H. (2010). Group-based parent-training programmes for improving emotional and behavioural adjustment in children from birth to three years old. *Cochrane Database of Systematic Reviews, 17*(3), CD003680.

Barlow, J., Bergman, H., Kornør, H., Wei, Y., & Bennett, C. (2016). Group-based parent training programmes for improving emotional and behavioural adjustment in young children. *The Cochrane Library.*

Berzins, L. G., & Trestman, R. L. (2004). The development and implementation of dialectical behavior therapy in forensic settings. *International Journal of Forensic Mental Health, 3*(1), 93–103. doi:http://dx.doi.org/10.1080/14999013.2004.10471199

Candelaria, A. M., Fedewa, A. L., & Ahn, S. (2012). The effects of anger management on children's social and emotional outcomes: A meta-analysis. *School Psychology International, 33*(6), 596–614.

Chamberlain, P., & Smith, D. K. (2005). Multidimensional treatment foster care: A community solution for boys and girls referred from juvenile justice. In E. D. Hibbs & P.S. Jensen (Eds.), *Psychosocial treatments for child and adolescent disorders: Empirically based strategies for clinical practice* (pp. 557–574). Washington, DC: American Psychological Association.

Clark, M. D., Walters, S., Gingerich, R., & Meltzer, M. (2006). Motivational interviewing for probation officers: Tipping the balance toward change. *Federal Probation, 70*, 38–44.

Colton, M., Vanstone, M., & Walby, C. (2002). Victimization, care and justice: Reflections on the experiences of victims/survivors involved in large-scale historical investigations of child sexual abuse in residential institutions. *British Journal of Social Work, 32*(5), 541–551.

Connor, D., Carlson, G., Chang, K., Daniolos, P., Ferziger, R., Findling, R., . . . Plattner, B. (2006). Juvenile maladaptive aggression: A review of prevention, treatment, and service configuration and a proposed research agenda. *Journal of Clinical Psychiatry, 67*(5), 808–820.

Connor, D. F., Glatt, S. J., Lopez, I. D., Jackson, D., & Melloni, R. H. (2002). Psychopharmacology and aggression. I: A meta-analysis of stimulant effects on overt/covert aggression–related behaviors in ADHD. *Journal of the American Academy of Child & Adolescent Psychiatry, 41*(3), 253–261.

Connor, D. F., Ozbayrak, K. R., Kusiak, K. A., Caponi, A. B., & Melloni, R. H. (1997). Combined pharmacotherapy in children and adolescents in a residential treatment center. *Journal of the American Academy of Child & Adolescent Psychiatry, 36*(2), 248–262.

Cunningham, R. M., Chermack, S. T., Zimmerman, M. A., Shope, J. T., Bingham, C. R., Blow, F. C., & Walton, M. A. (2012). Brief motivational interviewing intervention for peer violence and alcohol use in teens: One-year follow-up. *Pediatrics, 129*(6), 1083–1090.

Dakof, G. A., Henderson, C. E., Rowe, C. L., Boustani, M., Greenbaum, P. E., Wang, W., . . . Liddle, H. A. (2015). A randomized clinical trial of family therapy in juvenile drug court. *Journal of Family Psychology, 29*(2), 232.

Deković, M., Asscher, J. J., Manders, W. A., Prins, P. J., & van der Laan, P. (2012). Within-intervention change: mediators of intervention effects during multisystemic therapy. *Journal of Consulting and Clinical Psychology, 80*(4), 574–587.

De Swart, J. J. W., Van den Broek, H., Stams, G. J. J. M., Asscher, J. J., Van der Laan, P. H., Holsbrink-Engels, G. A., & Van der Helm, G. H. P. (2012). The effectiveness of institutional youth care over the past three decades: A meta-analysis. *Children and Youth Services Review, 34*(9), 1818–1824.

Devries, K. M., Knight, L., Child, J. C., Mirembe, A., Nakuti, J., Jones, R., . . . Parkes, J. (2015). The Good School Toolkit for reducing physical violence from school staff to primary school students: A cluster-randomised controlled trial in Uganda. *The Lancet Global Health, 3*(7), e378–e386.

Dishion, T. J., McCord, J., & Poulin, F. (1999). When interventions harm: Peer groups and problem behavior. *American Psychologist, 54*(9), 755–764.

Dodge, K. A., Malone, P. S., Lansford, J. E., Sorbring, E., Skinner, A. T., Tapanya, S., . . . Al-Hassan, S. M. (2015). Hostile attributional bias and aggressive behavior in global context. *Proceedings of the National Academy of Sciences, 112*(30), 9310–9315.

Enoch, M.-A., Kitzman, H., Smith, J. A., Anson, E., Hodgkinson, C. A., Goldman, D., & Olds, D. L. (2016). A prospective cohort study of influences on externalizing behaviors across childhood: Results from a nurse home visiting randomized controlled trial. *Journal of the American Academy of Child & Adolescent Psychiatry, 55*(5), 376–382.

Epstein, R. A., Fonnesbeck, C., Potter, S., Rizzone, K. H., & McPheeters, M. (2015). Psychosocial interventions for child disruptive behaviors: A meta-analysis. *Pediatrics, 136*(5), 2015–2577.

Gadow, K. D., Arnold, L. E., Molina, B. S., Findling, R. L., Bukstein, O. G., Brown, N. V., . . . Kipp, H. L. (2014). Risperidone added to parent training and stimulant medication: Effects on attention-deficit/hyperactivity disorder, oppositional defiant disorder, conduct disorder, and peer aggression. *Journal of the American Academy of Child & Adolescent Psychiatry, 53*(9), 948–959.

Garland, A. F., Hawley, K. M., Brookman-Frazee, L., & Hurlburt, M. S. (2008). Identifying common elements of evidence-based psychosocial treatments for children's disruptive behavior problems. *Journal of the American Academy of Child & Adolescent Psychiatry, 47*(5), 505–514.

Goodman, A. (2006). *The story of David Olds and the nurse home visiting program.* Princeton, NJ: Robert Wood Johnson Foundation.

Gorman, D. A., Gardner, D. M., Murphy, A. L., Feldman, M., Bélanger, S. A., Steele, M. M., . . . Soper, P. R. (2015). Canadian guidelines on pharmacotherapy for disruptive and aggressive behaviour in children and adolescents with attention-deficit hyperactivity disorder, opposi-tional defiant disorder, or conduct disorder. *The Canadian Journal of Psychiatry*, 60(2), 62–76.

Grant, J. E., & Leppink, E. W. (2015). Choosing a treatment for disruptive, impulse-control, and conduct disorders: Limited evidence, no approved drugs to guide treatment. *Current Psychiatry*, 14(1), 28–36.

Harper, R., & Hardy, S. (2000). Research note. An evaluation of motivational interviewing as a method of intervention with clients in a probation setting. *British Journal of Social Work*, 30(3), 393–400.

Hawes, D. J., & Dadds, M. R. (2005). The treatment of conduct problems in children with callous-unemotional traits. *Journal of Consulting and Clinical Psychology*, 73(4), 737–741.

Hawes, D. J., Price, M. J., & Dadds, M. R. (2014). Callous-unemotional traits and the treatment of conduct problems in childhood and adolescence: A comprehensive review. *Clinical Child and Family Psychology Review*, 17(3), 248–267.

Henggeler, S. W. (2012). Multisystemic therapy: Clinical foundations and research outcomes. *Psychosocial Intervention*, 21(2), 181–193.

Henggeler, S. W., Schoenwald, S. K., Borduin, C. M., Rowland, M. D., & Cunningham, P. B. (2009). *Multisystemic therapy for antisocial behavior in children and adolescents.* New York: Guilford Press.

Henggeler, S. W., & Sheidow, A. J. (2012). Empirically supported family-based treatments for conduct disorder and delinquency in adolescents. *Journal of Marital and Family Therapy*, 38(1), 30–58.

Hyde, L. W., Waller, R., Trentacosta, C. J., Shaw, D. S., Neiderhiser, J. M., Ganiban, J. M., . . . & Leve, L. D. (2016). Heritable and nonheritable pathways to early callous-unemotional behaviors. *American Journal of Psychiatry*, 173(9), 903–910.

James, S., Alemi, Q., Zepeda, V. (2013). Effectiveness and implementation of evidence-based prac-tices in residential care settings. *Children and Youth Services Review*, 35, 642–656.

Jensen, P. S., Youngstrom, E. A., Steiner, H., Findling, R. L., Meyer, R. E., Malone, R. P., . . . Blair, J. (2007). Consensus report on impulsive aggression as a symptom across diagnostic catego-ries in child psychiatry: Implications for medication studies. *Journal of the American Academy of Child & Adolescent Psychiatry*, 46(3), 309–322.

Kersten, L., Prätzlich, M., Mannstadt, S., Ackermann, K., Kohls, G., Oldenhof, H., . . . Popma, A. (2016). START NOW—a comprehensive skills training programme for female adolescents with oppositional defiant and conduct disorders: Study protocol for a cluster-randomised controlled trial. *Trials*, 17(1), 568.

Klein, R. G., Abikoff, H., Klass, E., Ganeles, D., Seese, L. M., & Pollack, S. (1997). Clinical efficacy of methylphenidate in conduct disorder with and without attention deficit hyperactivity dis-order. *Archives of General Psychiatry*, 54(12), 1073–1080.

Kochanska, G. (1997). Multiple pathways to conscience for children with different tempera-ments: from toddlerhood to age 5. *Developmental psychology*, 33(2), 228.

Kolko, D. J., & Pardini, D. A. (2010). ODD dimensions, ADHD, and callous–unemotional traits as predictors of treatment response in children with disruptive behavior disorders. *Journal of Abnormal Psychology*, 119(4), 713–725.

Linehan, M. M. (1993). *Cognitive-behavioral treatment of borderline personality disorder.* New York: Guilford Press.

Lipton, D., Martinson, R., & Wilks, J. (1975). *The effectiveness of correctional treatment: A survey of treatment evaluation studies.* New York: Praeger.

Lochman, J. E., Curry, J. F., Dane, H., & Ellis, M. (2001). The Anger Coping Program: An empiri-cally-supported treatment for aggressive children. *Residential Treatment for Children & Youth*, 18(3), 63–73.

Lochman, J. E., & Wells, K. C. (2002). The Coping Power program at the middle-school tran-sition: universal and indicated prevention effects. *Psychology of Addictive Behaviors*, 16(4S), S40.

Lochman, J. E., & Wells, K. C. (2003). Effectiveness of the Coping Power Program and of class-room intervention with aggressive children: Outcomes at a 1-year follow-up. *Behavior Therapy, 34*(4), 493–515.

Lochman, J. E., & Wells, K. C. (2004). The coping power program for preadolescent aggressive boys and their parents: outcome effects at the 1-year follow-up. *Journal of consulting and clinical psychology, 72*(4), 571.

Maughan, B., Rowe, R., Messer, J., Goodman, R., & Meltzer, H. (2004). Conduct disorder and oppositional defiant disorder in a national sample: Developmental epidemiology. *Journal of Child Psychology and Psychiatry, 45*(3), 609–621.

McCann, R. A., Ball, E. M., & Ivanoff, A. (2000). DBT with an inpatient forensic population: The CMHIP forensic model. *Cognitive and Behavioral Practice, 7*(4), 447–456.

Menting, J. G., Whittaker, J., Margetts, M. B., Whittaker, L. J., Kong, G. K.-W., Smith, B. J., . . . Jiráček, J. (2013). How insulin engages its primary binding site on the insulin receptor. *Nature, 493*(7431), 241–245.

Michelson, D., Davenport, C., Dretzke, J., Barlow, J., & Day, C. (2013). Do evidence-based interventions work when tested in the "real world?" A systematic review and meta-analysis of parent management training for the treatment of child disruptive behavior. *Clinical Child and Family Psychology Review, 16*(1), 18–34.

Miller, W. R., & Rollnick, S. (2012). *Motivational interviewing: Helping people change.* New York: Guilford Press.

National Institute for Clinical Excellence. (2013). Antisocial behaviour and conduct disorders in children and young people: recognition, intervention and management. *NICE Clinical Guideline 158.*

Padhy, R., Saxena, K., Remsing, L., Huemer, J., Plattner, B., & Steiner, H. (2011). Symptomatic response to divalproex in subtypes of conduct disorder. *Child Psychiatry & Human Development, 42*(5), 584–593.

Pappadopulos, E., MacIntyre, J. C., Crismon, M. L., Findling, R. L., Malone, R. P., Derivan, A., . . . Schur, S. B. (2003). Treatment recommendations for the use of antipsychotics for aggressive youth (TRAAY). Part II. *Journal of the American Academy of Child & Adolescent Psychiatry, 42*(2), 145–161.

Pappadopulos, E., Woolston, S., Chait, A., Perkins, M., Connor, D. F., & Jensen, P. S. (2006). Pharmacotherapy of aggression in children and adolescents: Efficacy and effect size. *Journal of the Canadian Academy of Child and Adolescent Psychiatry 5*(1), 27–39.

Pringsheim, T., Hirsch, L., Gardner, D., & Gorman, D. A. (2015a). The pharmacological management of oppositional behaviour, conduct problems, and aggression in children and adolescents with attention-deficit hyperactivity disorder, oppositional defiant disorder, and conduct disorder: A systematic review and meta-analysis. Part 1: Psychostimulants, alpha-2 agonists, and atomoxetine. *The Canadian Journal of Psychiatry, 60*(2), 42–51.

Pringsheim, T., Hirsch, L., Gardner, D., & Gorman, D. A. (2015b). The pharmacological management of oppositional behaviour, conduct problems, and aggression in children and adolescents with attention-deficit hyperactivity disorder, oppositional defiant disorder, and conduct disorder: A systematic review and meta-analysis. Part 2: Antipsychotics and traditional mood stabilizers. *The Canadian Journal of Psychiatry, 60*(2), 52–61.

Puzzanchera, C. (2013). *Juvenile arrests 2010.* Juvenile offenders and victims: National reports series. Washington, DC: Office of Juvenile Justice & Delinquency Prevention.

Quinn, A., & Shera, W. (2009). Evidence-based practice in group work with incarcerated youth. *International Journal of Law and Psychiatry, 32*(5), 288–293.

Ruths, S., & Steiner, H. (2004). Psychopharmacologic treatment of aggression in children and adolescents. *Pediatric Annals, 33*(5), 318–327.

Sanders, M. R., Kirby, J. N., Tellegen, C. L., & Day, J. J. (2014). The Triple P-Positive parenting program: A systematic review and meta-analysis of a multi-level system of parenting support. *Clinical Psychology Review, 34*(4), 337–357.

Sawyer, A. M., & Borduin, C. M. (2011). Effects of multisystemic therapy through midlife: a 21.9-year follow-up to a randomized clinical trial with serious and violent juvenile offenders. *Journal of Consulting and Clinical Psychology, 79*(5), 643.

Sawyer, A. M., Borduin, C. M., & Dopp, A. R. (2015). Long-term effects of prevention and treatment on youth antisocial behavior: A meta-analysis. *Clinical psychology Review, 42*, 130–144.

Saxena, K., Chang, K., & Steiner, H. (2006). Treatment of aggression with risperidone in children and adolescents with bipolar disorder: A case series. *Bipolar Disorders, 8*(4), 405–410.

Saxena, K., Howe, M., Simeonova, D., Steiner, H., & Chang, K. (2006). Divalproex sodium reduces overall aggression in youth at high risk for bipolar disorder. *Journal of Child & Adolescent Psychopharmacology, 16*(3), 252–259.

Saxena, K., Silverman, M. A., Chang, K., Khanzode, L., & Steiner, H. (2005). Baseline predictors of response to divalproex in conduct disorder. *Journal of Clinical Psychiatry, 66*(12), 1541–1548.

Schwartz, S., & Correll, C. U. (2014). Efficacy and safety of atomoxetine in children and adolescents with attention-deficit/hyperactivity disorder: Results from a comprehensive meta-analysis and metaregression. *Journal of the American Academy of Child & Adolescent Psychiatry, 53*(2), 174–187.

Scott, S., & Dadds, M. R. (2009). Practitioner review: When parent training doesn't work: Theory-driven clinical strategies. *Journal of Child Psychology and Psychiatry, 50*(12), 1441–1450.

Somech, L. Y., & Elizur, Y. (2012). Promoting self-regulation and cooperation in pre-kindergarten children with conduct problems: A randomized controlled trial. *Journal of the American Academy of Child & Adolescent Psychiatry, 51*(4), 412–422.

Spencer, T. J., Abikoff, H. B., Connor, D. F., Biederman, J., Pliszka, S. R., Boellner, S., . . . Pratt, R. (2006). Efficacy and safety of mixed amphetamine salts extended release (adderall XR) in the management of oppositional defiant disorder with or without comorbid attention-deficit/hyperactivity disorder in school-aged children and adolescents: A 4-week, multicenter, randomized, double-blind, parallel-group, placebo-controlled, forced-dose-escalation study. *Clinical Therapeutics, 28*(3), 402–418.

Spivack, G., Platt, J. J., & Shure, M. B. (1976). *The problem-solving approach to adjustment.* San Francisco: Jossey-Bass Publishers.

Stadler, C., Grasmann, D., Fegert, J. M., Holtmann, M., Poustka, F., & Schmeck, K. (2008). Heart rate and treatment effect in children with disruptive behavior disorders. *Child Psychiatry and Human Development, 39*(3), 299–309.

Stedman, T. L. (2006). *Stedman's medical dictionary.* Baltimore: Lippincott Williams & Wilkins.

Stein, L. A., Stein, L., Colby, S. M., Barnett, N. P., Monti, P. M., Golembeske, C., & Lebeau-Craven, R. (2006). Effects of motivational interviewing for incarcerated adolescents on driving under the influence after release. *American Journal on Addictions, 15*(Suppl. 1), 50–57.

Steiner, H. (2004). *Handbook of mental health interventions in children and adolescents: An integrated developmental approach.* San Francisco: Jossey-Bass.

Steiner, H., & Karnik, N. S. (2009). Integrated treatment of aggression in the context of ADHD in children refractory to stimulant monotherapy: A window into the future of child psychopharmacology. *The American Journal of Psychiatry, 166*(12), 1315–1317.

Steiner, H., Petersen, M. L., Saxena, K., Ford, S., & Matthews, Z. (2003). Divalproex sodium for the treatment of conduct disorder: A randomized controlled clinical trial. *Journal of Clinical Psychiatry, 64*(10), 1183–1191.

Steiner, H., & Remsing, L. (2007). Practice parameter for the assessment and treatment of children and adolescents with oppositional defiant disorder. *Journal of the American Academy of Child & Adolescent Psychiatry, 46*(1), 126–141.

Steiner, H., Saxena, K. S., Carrion, V., Khanzode, L. A., Silverman, M., & Chang, K. (2007). Divalproex sodium for the treatment of PTSD and conduct disordered youth: A pilot randomized controlled clinical trial. *Child Psychiatry and Human Development, 38*(3), 183–193.

van der Stouwe, T., Asscher, J. J., Stams, G. J. J., Deković, M., & van der Laan, P. H. (2014). The effectiveness of Multisystemic Therapy (MST): A meta-analysis. *Clinical Psychology Review, 34*(6), 468–481.

Viding, E., Fontaine, N. M., & McCrory, E. J. (2012). Antisocial behaviour in children with and without callous-unemotional traits. *Journal of the Royal Society of Medicine, 105*(5), 195–200.

Wagner, D. V., Borduin, C. M., Sawyer, A. M., & Dopp, A. R. (2014). Long-term prevention of criminality in siblings of serious and violent juvenile offenders: A 25-year follow-up to a randomized clinical trial of multisystemic therapy. *Journal of Consulting and Clinical Psychology, 82*(3), 492–499.

Waller, R., Gardner, F., & Hyde, L. W. (2013). What are the associations between parenting, callous–unemotional traits, and antisocial behavior in youth? A systematic review of evidence. *Clinical Psychology Review, 33*(4), 593–608.

Waschbusch, D. A., Carrey, N. J., Willoughby, M. T., King, S., & Andrade, B. F. (2007). Effects of methylphenidate and behavior modification on the social and academic behavior of children with disruptive behavior disorders: The moderating role of callous/unemotional traits. *Journal of Clinical Child and Adolescent Psychology, 36*(4), 629–644.

Webster-Stratton, C., Jamila Reid, M., & Stoolmiller, M. (2008). Preventing conduct problems and improving school readiness: Evaluation of the incredible years teacher and child training programs in high-risk schools. *Journal of Child Psychology and Psychiatry, 49*(5), 471–488.

Wilkinson, S., Waller, R., & Viding, E. (2015). Practitioner review: Involving young people with callous unemotional traits in treatment–does it work? A systematic review. *Journal of Child Psychology and Psychiatry, 57*(5), 552–565.

6

Forensic Implications
in Disruptive Behavior Disorders

6.1 Definitions and Introduction

In this chapter, we discuss the considerable overlap that exists between youth with disruptive behavior disorders (DBDs) and the juvenile justice system. In order to prime readers who are not familiar with the juvenile courts and/or forensic psychiatry, we begin by providing some basic definitions. These are followed by a summary of some of the landmark legal cases that have shaped the ways that youth in our juvenile justice system are treated. Next, we review how recent findings form developmental neuroscience, in particular how the concept of "developmental immaturity" has influenced thinking in our field and the juvenile courts. We then progress to a discussion of juvenile desistance and the important work of Teplin and colleagues (2002, 2013), looking at psychopathology among incarcerated youth. From here we briefly review subtypes of juvenile offenders and sociodemographic variables related to juvenile delinquency, including a discussion of gender and the growing rates at which young women are entering the juvenile justice system. We describe some of the structured tools that forensic psychiatrists and psychologists use when performing violence and/or sexual violence risk assessments on juvenile justice involved youth. We also discuss the implications that a young person's personality traits and aggression profile may have when professionals are asked to estimate his or her amenability to treatment and/or risk of committing future violent acts. We conclude by reviewing some of the treatment approaches that have been designed specifically for juvenile justice involved youth with conduct problems followed by a discussion of some ethical issues pertinent to the diagnosis, treatment, and forensic evaluation of such youth.

Forensic: "Pertaining or applicable to personal injury, murder, and other legal proceedings" (Stedman, 2006).

Forensic medicine: "the relation and application of medical facts to legal matters" (Stedman, 2006).

Forensic psychiatry: "the application of psychiatry in courts of law, e.g., in determinations for commitment, competency, fitness to stand trial, responsibility for crime" (Stedman, 2006).

A more comprehensive definition of forensic psychiatry is provided by the American Academy of Psychiatry and the Law (AAPL) as follows:

> Forensic psychiatry is a medical subspecialty that includes research and clinical practice in the many areas in which psychiatry is applied to legal issues. While some forensic psychiatrists may specialize exclusively in legal issues, almost all psychiatrists may, at some point, have to work within one of the many areas in which the mental health and legal system overlap. AAPL welcomes both the forensic specialist and the general psychiatrist who seeks information and professional support in those domains in which psychiatry and the law share a common boundary. These include:
>
> - Violence
> - Criminal responsibility
> - Competence, civil and criminal
> - Child custody and visitation
> - Psychic injury
> - Mental disability
> - Malpractice
> - Confidentiality
> - Involuntary treatment
> - Correctional psychiatry
> - Juvenile justice
> - Ethics and human rights
>   (AAPL, 2014)

Expert witness: "a witness (as a medical specialist) who by virtue of special knowledge, skill, training, or experience is qualified to provide testimony to aid the factfinder in matters that exceed the common knowledge of ordinary people" (Merriam-Webster, 2006).

Culpable: "deserving condemnation or blame as wrong or harmful" (Merriam-Webster, 2006).

Finally, for readers who are wondering who we are and why we feel passionate about our decision to create a chapter focusing on the overlap between DBDs and juvenile justice involved youth, we provide a bit of background information.

All of the authors of this text have experience diagnosing, treating, and performing forensic evaluations and/or conducting research on adults and youth in the
justice systems. The main author of this book, Dr. Hans Steiner, is the director of
Stanford University's Program in Psychiatry and the Law within the Department
of Psychiatry and Behavioral Sciences. Dr. Steiner has spent his academic and
clinical career working with adolescents and young adults in adult correctional
settings. He has conducted studies for the National Institute of Justice (NIJ)
in juvenile justice and adult settings, written papers on improving standards
of care for incarcerated youth for national organizations, and provided expert
consultation on these topics to California governors. Dr. Steiner has also served
as an expert witness more than 200 civil and criminal cases, many of which
have involved youth with severe behavior problems. Dr. Whitney Daniels is a
Stanford University psychiatrist boarded in both general and child and adolescent psychiatry. Dr. Daniels serves as assistant director of Stanford's Program
in Psychiatry and the Law. She has a wealth of experience treating, evaluating,
and writing about youth with DBDs and juvenile justice system involvement.
Like Dr. Daniels, Dr. Mike Kelly is an assistant director of Stanford's Program
in Psychiatry and the Law. Dr. Kelly is also the director of training for Stanford's
burgeoning forensic psychiatry fellowship program. Dr. Kelly is boarded in general, child and adolescent, and forensic psychiatry. In addition to writing on the
topic of DBDs and attention deficit hyperactivity disorder (ADHD), Dr. Kelly
has worked in a variety of correctional, state hospital, and community settings
with court-involved children and adults. Dr. Christina Stadler is a professor at
the Kinder und Jugendlichen Psychiatrie Klinik of the University of Basel. She
is the director of the Department of Research at the Diagnostic and Therapeutic
Day Klinik. Her research expertise is in DBDs. Dr. Stadler is a frequent presenter
at national and international professional meetings. She has published more
than 75 scientific papers on youth with DBDs, ADHD, and related problems
with impulse control. Next we provide some statistics on the overlap between
juvenile justice involved youth and DBDs.

6.2 DBDs and Juvenile Justice Involved Youth

Historically, a large percentage of youth involved in the juvenile justice system
have met *Diagnostic and Statistical Manual of Mental Disorders* (DSM) criteria for
a DBD. Teplin, Abram, McClelland, Dulcan, and Mericle (2002) have estimated
that roughly two-thirds of males and nearly 74% of females in juvenile detention meet criteria for at least one or more psychiatric disorders. They also found
that approximately 41% of the males and 46% of females in juvenile detention
met criteria for a DBD. It is worth noting that some studies that have looked

exclusively at juvenile delinquents who were postadjudication have indicated that the percentages of psychiatric disorders, including DBDs, is even greater than Teplin et al.'s work suggests (Bauer et al., 2011; Celio, Karnik, & Steiner, 2006; Niranjan, Karnik, McMullin, & Steiner, 2006; Karnik et al., 2009; Karnik et al., 2010; Karnik & Steiner, 2007; Kaszynski et al., 2014; Plattner et al., 2012; Plattner et al., 2007; Plattner et al., 2009; Steiner et al., 2011). A number of studies, some of which we delve into later in this chapter, have looked specifically at these disorders and aggression in the juvenile justice population. As the literature cited attests, we can confidently state that the advancements made in understanding DBDs has great potential for contributing to a more rational approach to child and adolescent forensic psychiatry.

In chapter 1 we summarized shifts that occurred in America around the turn of the last century that had a major impact on its justice system. Most notably, American courts became more cognizant of youths' age when making decisions regarding alleged criminal offenses, which helped lead to the development of a formal juvenile justice system—a juvenile justice system intended to help youth regain a positive developmental course through some combination of psychosocial treatment, parental education, and community level intervention. We next summarize some cases that are particularly relevant to juvenile delinquency, DBDs, and young people's potential for redemption in the eyes of the US justice system.

6.2.1 *IN RE GAULT* (1967)

The first case addresses the important question of whether juveniles who are charged with a crime should be afforded procedural due process rights akin to adult defendants. (note that "procedural due process" refers to fair procedures to which the government must adhere before taking away someone's life, liberty, or property). During the summer of 1964 a 15-year-old boy from Gila County, Arizona, named Gerald Gault was hanging out at home with a friend, Ronald Lewis. Gerald was already on probation for an incident in which he reportedly accompanied another boy who stole a wallet from a woman's purse. In a fit of adolescent boredom, Gerald and Ronald allegedly prank-called a neighbor, Ms. Ora Cook, making some lewd comments. For example, the callers supposedly asked Ms. Cook, "Do you have big bombers?" and "Are your cherries ripe today?" None too pleased, an angry Ms. Cook recognized one of the voices on the line as Gerald's and called the Gila County Sheriff to file a complaint. What happened next is perhaps the most well-documented overreaction to a prank call in US history. Gerald and Ronald were taken into custody by the county sheriff and immediately transported to the Children's Detention Home located in Gila County. Neither boys' parents were notified that their sons had been taken into custody, and multiple court hearings were held without the boys being provided any advance warning or legal representation. To make matters worse, there were not even transcripts of the hearings that led to Gerald being committed to a trade school until the age of 21. Had Gerald and his buddy Ronald been adults at the time of their alleged prank call, the maximum penalties in this case would have been $50 with up to two months in county jail.

When Gerald's mother returned home from work and found out what was happening, she traveled to the Children's Detention Home but was not allowed to speak to her son. Understandably upset, Gerald's parents filed a petition of habeas corpus (i.e., a request for the court to consider Gerald's detention unlawful). Gerald's petition for habeas corpus was dismissed by the Superior Court of Arizona and later by the Arizona Supreme Court. Gerald's case was appealed to the US Supreme Court, which granted certiorari (i.e., the US Supreme Court agreed to review the lower courts' decisions). In 1967 the court agreed with Gerald and his parents when it ruled that that the lower courts' decisions were unconstitutional and that juveniles are entitled to procedural safeguards under the Due Process Clause of the Fourteenth Amendment to the US Constitution. The safeguards that Gerald and Ronald were entitled to include the right to receive a written notice of charges, the right to legal counsel, and the right to confront witnesses in their own defense. The Gault decision was an important legal reform in that it specified the types of due process protections that youth should be able to rely upon in the juvenile justice system. *In re Gault* marked a serious step forward in how young people were supposed to be adjudicated, at least in theory, if not always in actual practice.

6.2.2 *ROPER V. SIMMONS* (2005)

Our next case addressed the question of whether it is unconstitutional to execute someone who commits a capital crime while still a minor. Christopher Simmons, a 17-year-old Missouri teen, conspired to "murder someone" before he turned 18. In order to act out his fantasy, Christopher enlisted the help of two younger boys, one of whom had misgivings and bailed on their plan. During the early morning hours of September 9, 1993, Christopher and a 15-year-old accomplice, Charles Benjamin, broke into the home of 46-year-old wife and mother Mrs. Shirley Crook. Mrs. Crook's husband was away on a fishing trip when Christopher and Charles snuck into her home. Christopher later reported that he experienced some misgivings about the plan until he recognized Mrs. Crook as the woman he had been involved with in a minor traffic accident the previous year. Christopher and Benjamin subsequently bound Mrs. Crook's hands behind her back, taped her eyes and mouth shut with duct tape, and wrapped her in blankets fastened around her with leather straps and electrical cord. The boys used Mrs. Crook's minivan to drive her to a railroad trestle over the Meramec River where Christopher tossed her into the water while she was fully conscious. Christopher bragged about the killing to peers afterward and was eventually apprehended by police.

Christopher was charged as an adult for killing Mrs. Crook, convicted, and sentenced to death by a trial court. Christopher's case was appealed to the Missouri Supreme Court, which agreed with trial court's decision. A second appeal was filed with the Missouri Supreme Court, which disagreed with the lower court's decisions based in part on the "evolving standards of decency" argument used by the US Supreme Court to prohibit the execution of mentally retarded individuals in case of *Atkins v. Virginia* (2002). The case was then appealed to the US Supreme Court, which held (i.e., ruled) that executing someone who committed a capital crime while still a minor was a violation of said minor's rights under the Eighth and Fourteenth Amendments. The court cited the work of Dr. Laurence Steinberg pertaining to the concept of "developmental immaturity," which we discuss in detail later in this chapter, and its role as a mitigating factor (i.e., evidence about the defendant and/or circumstances of a crime that leads to reductions in the criminal charges or sentence).

Sentencing minors to death for capital crimes raises important ethical concerns given the lack of certitude in the developmental psychopathology literature on our ability to predict which youth will go on to become bona fide psychopaths, the mitigating role that developmental immaturity can play for minors well into their teens, and the apparent inequities in the criminal justice system's application of the death penalty along racial/ethnic, socioeconomic, and geographic lines (Alesina & La Ferrara, 2014; Bright, 1994, 2008, 2014; Frick, Kimonis, Dandreaux, & Farell, 2003; Johnson & Johnson, 2001; Kleck, 1981; Levinson, Smith, & Young, 2014; Steinberg & Scott, 2003). In our view, despite the calculated, callous, and horrific nature of Mr. Simmons' crime, the US Supreme Court rightly prohibited sentencing individuals who committed capital crimes as minors to death in *Roper v. Simmons*.

6.2.3 *GRAHAM V. FLORIDA* (2010)

In 2010 the case of *Graham v. Florida* came before the US Supreme Court. This case examined whether the Eighth Amendment and its provision against cruel and unusual punishment made it unconstitutional to sentence a minor to life without the possibility of parole for crimes that did not include homicide. In the year 2003, at the age of 16, Terrance Graham and two other young men attempted to rob a Jacksonville, Florida, barbecue restaurant. Terrance was apprehended and charged as an adult for charges that included burglary with assault, battery, and attempted armed robbery. Terrance pleaded guilty and was ultimately placed on probation. Terrance was arrested again six months later in connection with an alleged home invasion and robbery. A Florida trial court ultimately found Terrance guilty of a variety of charges, and he was given the maximum possible sentence in light of what the court described as an "escalating pattern of criminal conduct." Unfortunately, after all of Terrance's sentences were added up, he was essentially given a life sentence by the trial court due to the fact that Florida had done away with its parole system. Terrance's sentences were upheld by Florida's First District Court of Appeals, and the Florida Supreme Court declined to review his case. However, the US Supreme Court agreed to review Terrance's case, and in an opinion issued by Justice Kennedy said, "The Constitution prohibits the imposition of a life without parole sentence on a juvenile offender who did not commit homicide." While the court held that states did not need to guarantee a juvenile offender's eventual release, they must "provide him or her some realistic opportunity to obtain release before the end of that term." We agree with the US Supreme Court's decision in *Graham v. Florida* because, from our developmental perspective, the extant literature indicates that courts should be mindful of the potential impact of a youth's developmental immaturity, absence of a fully formed character, and patterns of juvenile desistance, even among those who have committed violent crimes, when sentencing minors. The *Graham* decision making it unconstitutional to sentence minors who committed crimes other than murder to life without the possibility of parole set the stage for the final two UA Supreme Court cases we discuss in this section—two cases that, in our opinion, raise major ethical questions that our field must help address in the years to come.

6.2.4 MILLER V. ALABAMA (2012)

In 2012 the US Supreme Court ruled on whether it is constitutional to allow juvenile offenders to be sentenced to life without the possibility of parole. *Miller v. Alabama* was the conglomeration of two different cases involving 14-year-old boys charged with murder, Evan Miller from Alabama and Kuntrell Jackson from Arkansas. Both boys were charged as adults, convicted, and sentenced to life without the possibility of parole. Evan and Kuntrell's appeals in both states were unsuccessful, and the US Supreme Court agreed to review their cases. Relying heavily on the rationale put forth in the cases of *Roper v. Simmons* and *Graham v. Florida* decisions, the court ruled that the mandatory sentencing of juveniles to life without the possibility of parole constituted cruel and unusual punishment and was in violation of the Eighth Amendment. The court added that sentencing juveniles who have committed homicide was not inherently unconstitutional so long as certain factors such as "chronological age and its hallmark features—among them, immaturity, impetuosity, and failure to appreciate risks and consequences" were taken into account. Although we largely agree with the US Supreme Court's decision in *Miller v. Alabama*, in our view, this case raises serious ethical and legal questions that we attempt to shed more light on in our discussion of the next case.

6.2.5 *MONTGOMERY V. LOUISIANA* (2016)

Henry Montgomery was 17 years old in 1963 when he killed Charles Hurt, an East Baton Rouge Parish sheriff deputy, in the state of Louisiana. Henry was found guilty of murder and sentenced to life without the possibility of parole. Almost 50 years later, the US Supreme Court ruled in the case of *Miller v. Alabama* (2012) that mandatory life sentencing of minors without the possibility of parole was unconstitutional. In 2016 the US Supreme Court's ruling in the case of *Montgomery v. Louisiana* expanded and made retroactive its decision in *Miller v. Alabama*. The court also held that sentencing an individual who committed crimes while under the age of 18 (e.g., murder) to life without the possibility of parole is unconstitutional, unless said individual is found to be "irreparably corrupt" or "permanently incorrigible."

In essence, the US Supreme Court has decided that it is unconstitutional to sentence a minor to life without the possibility of parole unless said minor is, for all intents and purposes, unredeemable. We argue that such a loophole for sentencing minors to life without the possibility of parole raises important scientific and ethical questions. For example, what standard will courts, presumably with the assistance of mental health professionals, use to determine whether a juvenile is "irreparably corrupt" or "permanently incorrigible"? Might these labels become synonymous with youth described as having a "psychopathic personality" or possessing "callous–unemotional traits," or, in the language of the current version of the DSM, those who display "limited prosocial emotions"? For the sake of argument, let us assume that courts will be most likely to raise the issue of whether a juvenile is "irreparably corrupt" with those who possess callous–unemotional traits. Also, with what degree of certainty can mental health professionals comment on whether a minor is "irreparably corrupt"? In order to begin answering this question, we first need to find out what the literature has to say about the persistence of callous–unemotional traits over time.

A study by Kolko and Pardini (2010) found that callous–unemotional traits did not bear any discernible relation to outcomes three years after treatment. This study's findings are significant because they suggest that callous–unemotional traits may be malleable over time, which, if true, could have major treatment and legal implications. While a more recent meta-analysis showed that callous–unemotional traits are in fact associated with poorer treatment outcomes, the authors also concluded that certain parent training interventions can attenuate callous–unemotional traits, especially with early intervention (Hawes, Price, & Dadds, 2014). Furthermore, Frick and colleagues (2003, p. 733) put forth some interesting points about why we should use caution in predicting the likelihood that a youths' callous–unemotional traits will persist into adulthood. For example, Frick and colleagues succinctly point out that in accordance with a perspective put forth by Cicchetti and Rogosch (1996), "a hallmark of taking a developmental approach to understanding psychopathological conditions is that, as one attempts to understand the developmental processes that can lead to an outcome of interest, one should assume that the pathways are changeable" (Frick et al., 2003, p. 177). Data indicating that callous–unemotional traits during youth are not always predictive of adult psychopathy and are not necessarily impervious to treatment are a source of hope for treatment providers and a call for forensic psychiatrists and psychologists to exercise great caution and consideration before suggesting that a juvenile offender is "irreparably corrupt" or "permanently incorrigible."

Vignette

Mitchell was a 15-year-old boy with no formal psychiatric history who lived in a rural part of California's central valley. Mitchell was a decent student who had relatively few friends and was generally avoided by his peers. He lived with his mother and her boyfriend, both of whom used a variety of drugs and drank heavily. When Mitchell was a toddler he experienced extreme neglect and physical abuse at the hands of his mother and biological father, who were still together at that time. Around the age of 13 Mitchell began luring grade school children into an abandoned barn with the promise of candy. Mitchell started off fondling the younger children, but over time his sexual advances became more aggressive. Mitchell would tell his victims that they would get in trouble if anyone knew they had engaged in sexual activity together and that he would ultimately "kill" them if they talked. Around Mitchell's 15th birthday, he kidnapped two nine-year-old boys over the span of two weeks. Mitchell sexually assaulted, tortured, and then ultimately killed each boy. Mitchell stashed the boys' bodies under a pile of rocks in a nearby river before they were eventually discovered and he was arrested. Mitchell's evaluation was notable for a resting heart rate of 48 bpm, and he discussed his crimes in a matter-of-fact manner. At one point during the interview, Mitchell described the moment he killed one of his victims in graphic detail and flashed a slight smile. While it is impossible to know exactly what Mitchell was thinking or feeling at that time, he gave the impression that he derived pleasure from making others uncomfortable when he discussed his deeds. Mitchell was waived to adult court and received a lengthy sentence.

6.3 Culpability and Developmental Immaturity

An important consideration for courts when adjudicating minors relates to the concept of "developmental immaturity." This pioneering concept was developed by a variety of academics specializing in child development who include Drs. Laurence Steinberg, Elizabeth Cauffman, and Thomas Grisso, in addition to law professor Elizabeth Scott. These scholars have argued, and the authors of this text agree, that additional factors must be considered for youths who have committed or are accused of committing crimes. This is because youth are still developing decision-making capacities and tend to be susceptible to coercion and/or peer pressure, plus the fact that their personalities or "characters" are not yet fully formed. While there is no formally agreed-upon definition of "developmental immaturity," we broadly define it as functional limitations resulting from the incomplete development of a youth's cognitive ability, ability to function independently, decision-making ability, and/or ability to regulate his or her emotions.

A landmark paper by Grisso and colleagues (2003) looked specifically at the adjudicative competence (i.e., a minor's competence to stand trial) of over 900 adolescents in juvenile detention and in community settings and compared this with over 450 adults in county jails and the community. Grisso and colleagues found that young people ages 15 or below tended to perform more poorly than young adults on formal measures of their competence to stand trial. Additionally, teenagers tended to make choices about their cases (e.g., deciding whether to accept a plea bargain) that were largely influenced by their desire to comply with the perceived wishes of law enforcement at the expense of what was in their own best interests legally. Furthermore, younger teenagers tended to have difficulty grasping the implications and risks associated with legal decisions due to their immature thinking (Grisso et al., 2003).

At present, the US Supreme Court has not ruled on a standard for determining a juvenile's competence to stand trial. In his 2015 article titled "Eliminating the Competency Presumption in Juvenile Delinquency Cases," Tulane University Law School Clinical Professor David Katner argues for doing away with US courts' presumption that juveniles are competent for adjudication. In Katner's view, such a change would help our juvenile courts do a better job of considering the impact of developmental immaturity and high rates of mental illness among juvenile offenders, thereby moving us toward a model that prioritizes rehabilitation over the adjudication of minors. We suggest that in the absence of a national standard for determining juvenile defendants' adjudicative competence, mental health professionals who perform such evaluations need to remain appraised of the standards in their local jurisdiction and familiar with the literature on developmental immaturity.

Steinberg and Scott (2003) argued that juveniles should not be held to the same standards of criminal responsibility as adults because their decision-making capacity is diminished, they are less able to resist coercive influence, and their character is still undergoing change. Supporting this statement is a study performed by Cauffman and Steinberg (2000). Their study measured factors relevant to "maturity of judgment" in over 1,000 individuals between the ages of 12 and 48. Factors related to people's mature decision-making abilities included "responsibility" (e.g., self-reliance, sense of identity, self-esteem, level of pride in their work), "perspective" (e.g., ability to consider short- and long-term consequences, capacity to consider the perspective of others when making decisions), and "temperance" (e.g., impulse control and ability to control their aggression). Participants were asked to respond to a series of hypothetical questions pertaining to behaviors that had the potential to be risky and/or overtly antisocial. Cauffman and Steinberg found that participants tended to make more "socially responsible" decisions in young adulthood versus adolescence; however, this tendency did not increase in a meaningful way after participants reached the age of 19. In general, people who displayed higher degrees of responsibility, perspective, and temperance as described showed more maturity when making decisions regardless of age. That said, adolescents as a whole tended to score lower in these areas as compared to adults. This study was important because it was one of the first to address the question of whether youth should be held to the same standards of culpability as adults on an empirical basis rather than mere logical reasoning (Cauffman & Steinberg, 2000).

In 2012, child and adolescent forensic psychiatrist and director of the Psychiatry and the Law Service at Emory University Dr. Peter Ash published an article on 10 factors forensic psychiatrists can use as a guide when formulating opinions on the criminal culpability of adolescents. The factors that Ash describes in his article are based on the extant literature pertaining to adolescent development and antisocial behavior. Ash rightfully acknowledges the ambiguous nature methods courts and mental health professionals have used to formulate opinions on adolescent culpability. His paper also touches on the legal implications of a forensic evaluators findings. Although it is beyond the scope of this text to delve deeply into the details of how to assess criminal culpability in adolescents, a listing of the factors Ash recommends juvenile evaluators consider when assessing adolescent culpability (Box 6.1) provides a succinct outline to a thoughtful approach.

Box 6.1 **Factors to Consider in Assessing Adolescent Culpability**

1. Appreciation of wrongfulness
2. Ability to conform to law
3. Developmental course of aggression and impulsivity
4. Immaturity: IQ, psychosocial maturity, including time sense, susceptibility to peer pressure, risk taking, ability to empathize
5. Out-of-character action
6. Environmental circumstances
7. Peer group norms
8. Incomplete personality development
9. Mental illness
10. Reactive attitudes toward the offense

Source: Ash, P. (2012). But he knew it was wrong: Evaluating adolescent culpability. *Journal of the American Academy of Psychiatry and the Law Online*, 40(1), 21–32.)

6.4 Classifications of Juvenile Offenders: Criminal Typologies and Profiling

In our view, forensic evaluators cannot meaningfully understand youth based on their types of offenses no more than an auto mechanic can understand the inner workings of automobiles based on their paint schemes. As we have asserted throughout this book, juvenile delinquency and DBDs occur in a variety of social, familial, genetic, cognitive, and emotional contexts. From the delinquency literature, we know that, at least in the early stages of development, there are no "crime specialists." Categorizing juveniles according to the types of crimes they commit may serve important purposes for the process of adjudication, but such classification schemes has limited utility from a developmental psychopathology perspective (Steiner, Humphreys, & Redlich, 2001).

That said, an exception to these statements should be made with regard to emerging evidence for the utility of a typology for juvenile sex offenders. Recent research on juvenile sexual violence has found distinctions between "specialists" (i.e., youth that only commit sexual offenses) versus "generalists" (i.e., youth who commit sexual offenses in addition to other forms of violent crime). For instance, Chu and Thomas's (2010) study from Singapore investigated the criminal versatility (i.e., variety of types of crime committed) and recidivism among

156 adolescent boys who had committed sexual offenses. This study found that boys who had committed sexual offenses but no other types of violent crime were more likely to have victims from within their own families. However, boys who had committed both sexual offenses and other violent crimes had similar rates of sexual recidivism to those who had committed only sexual offenses. Not surprisingly, the youth who had engaged in both sexual offenses and other types of violent crime were overall more likely to violently reoffend. While this study provides interesting information about the increased likelihood of having inter-familial victims for adolescent boys who had engaged only in sexual offenses, it does not shed light on the heterogeneity within this group and who among them is most likely to reoffend.

A recent meta-analysis showed that the vast majority of adolescent sex offenders are generalists who are similar other types of violent juvenile offenders (Pullman & Seto, 2012). However, adolescent specialist sex offenders tend to have unique risk factors that include a history of childhood sexual abuse and/or maltreatment and unusual sexual interests. These data have implications for the types of treatment that may be beneficial for the generalists versus the specialists. These studies and others like it are encouraging in that they suggest the potential identifiable developmental pathways for becoming a specialist juvenile sex offender, similar to what is becoming known about juvenile psychopathy. Aside from some notable exceptions, classifying youth based on the types of offense they commit, at present, is of limited utility. We argue that the rapidly growing body of information the field has gained through advancements in developmental neuroscience has yet to be fully explored and made use of within the American juvenile justice system.

A 2012 study by Mulder, Vermunt, Brand, Bullens, and Marle from the Netherlands sought to determine if serious juvenile offenders can be divided into subgroups based on their type of offense and whether these subgroups differed in regard to risk factors that are predictive of recidivism. The study included over 1,100 "serious juvenile offenders" who were divided into the subgroups comprised of serious violent offenders, violent property offenders, property offenders, and sexual offenders. The violent property offenders subgroup were most likely to reoffend and tended to have more risk factors for recidivism, followed by the property offenders group. The sex offenders subgroup was least likely to reoffend. Interestingly, each of the four groups had different sets of risk factors that predicted the degree of recidivism (Mulder et al., 2012).

A limitation of this study was that it did not measure tendencies toward hot versus cold aggression (i.e., referred to earlier in this text as reactive/affective/defensive/impulsive [RADI] and proactive/instrumental/planned [PIP] aggression, respectively) and the presence of callous–unemotional traits among participants. It is worth noting that the two groups with the highest likelihood of recidivism, violent property offenders and property offenders, tended to score higher on measures designed to quantify a lack of conscience and insight. How might have the results of this study been different if participants were classified according to aggression profile and the presence of callous–unemotional traits? We argue that future research on the subtypes of juvenile offenders should be based on an approach that is sensitive to neurodevelopmental differences rather than categorizing behaviors (i.e., juvenile offenses) regardless of the context in which they occur.

The stated concerns about classifying juveniles according to types of offense is consistent with the adult literature on criminal profiling. For example, in the late 1970s, Groth, Burgess, and Holmstrom (1977) published a typology for three distinct types of rapists comprised of the "anger rapist," the "power rapist," and the "sadistic rapist." Additional offender typologies and models have been created over the years, including a "Power and Anger" model that has been utilized extensively in the United States by the Federal Bureau of Investigation (FBI; Hazelwood, 1987; Hazelwood, Ressler, Depue, & Douglas, 1995). A recent study from the United Kingdom used a sample comprised of 85 "stranger rapists" (i.e., rapists who did not know their victims or had met them just prior to the assault) to compare the ability of three different well-known offender profiling modes, including the Power and Anger FBI model with that of a multivariate regression approach that was based on a combination of crime scene behaviors to find out which of these approaches did a better job at predicting the offenders' previous convictions (Goodwill, Alison, & Beech, 2009). This study found that the multivariate approach based on certain crime scene behaviors was far superior to the three widely used profiling models. In general, the effectiveness of criminal profiling based on the types of crimes committed and crime scene characteristics has been the subject of much scrutiny and skepticism. Snook, Cullen, Bennell, Taylor, and Gendreau (2008) cite an abundance of evidence in arguing that criminal profiling in general lacks scientific support, and we agree.

A study by Plattner and colleagues (2012) showed that among 275 incarcerated teenage boys, those with alcohol use disorders, in absence of other substance use disorders, tended to commit more violent crime. Incarcerated boys with substance use disorders, other than an alcohol use disorder, tended to commit more drug-related crimes. The only other significant finding from this study was that detained boys without anxiety disorders were more likely to commit robbery. The lack of criminological types evident from this study reinforces the notion that social, familial, and biologic contexts, rather than diagnostic labels, are essential for understanding the roots of aggression and delinquent behavior (Plattner et al., 2012).

The studies cited and our findings in a report for the California Youth Authority (CYA) referenced throughout this chapter indicate that the overlap between psychopathology and criminological types is almost random. Thus we must be cognizant that when criminological types are being "treated" (i.e., rehabilitated and punished) within the juvenile justice system, it is not the same thing as medical and psychiatric treatment. Treatment in the psychiatric-medical context refers to the healing of a diagnosable condition, which may or may not lead to criminological rehabilitation. The specific and contrasting contributions of the juvenile justice systems approach to rehabilitation and the medical-psychiatric model's approach to treatment on the prognosis for juvenile delinquency is yet to be studied more carefully. For now, it is safe to assume that psychiatric treatment utilizes a set of tools (e.g., psychotherapy, medication, behavioral reinforcement, etc.) that are largely distinct from the "treatment," or rather, rehabilitative efforts, employed by the juvenile justice system, particularly for those in juvenile detention (e.g., institutionalization with associated behavioral incentives to progress towards release). It is likely that these two approaches often complement, or even augment, each other; however, we do not have enough data presently to make such proclamations with confidence. Simply stated, criminal profiling is an inexact science. Approaches to profiling and prescribing treatment based on the types of crime committed alone, devoid of developmental considerations, has serious flaws.

6.5 Juvenile Desistance

Desistance is a term used by criminologists to describe individuals who stop committing crimes and other antisocial acts. Interestingly, while everyone can agree on what the term means, there is a lot of variability in how researchers define and quantify desistance from crime. Given some of the gaps in our knowledge about juvenile desistance, Lussier, McCuish, and Corrado (2015) advocate for a "unified model of desistance" that accounts for the heterogeneity among juvenile offenders along a continuum that includes active criminality, the deceleration of criminal behavior, and termination of offending.

The Pathways to Desistance Study followed 1,354 "serious juvenile offenders" (1,170 males and 184 females) between the ages of 14 and 18 during a span of seven years (Mulvey, 2011). Serious juvenile offenders in this study were defined as youth who had been found guilty of one or more serious violent crimes, property offenses, or drug offenses. According Dr. Edward Mulvey's concise summary of the Pathways to Desistance Study, the vast majority of adolescents who commit felonies stop or reduce their offending over time. In fact, 91.5% of participants reported reductions in criminal behavior over the first three years following their court involvement. Also, longer stays in juvenile detention were not shown to reduce the likelihood of recidivism, with some increasing their frequency of criminal behavior after incarceration. Community-based supervision following incarceration was shown to be an effective means of reducing recidivism adolescents who have committed serious crimes. Substance abuse treatment, particularly treatment that lasted at least 90 days and included family participation, resulted in substantial drops in marijuana use, alcohol use, and offending for up to six months posttreatment.

While the Pathways to Desistance Study provides important, and some-what reassuring, information on serious juvenile offenders, it is not without limitations. For instance, much of the information gathered in this study was based on participants' self-report. The extent to which participants may have been incentivized to underreport their level of criminal behavior is not clear. In addition, this study's focus on primarily male "serious juvenile offenders" does not reflect the heterogeneity within the juvenile justice population. Furthermore, this study did not consider aggression profiles when monitoring which youth were most likely to offend. Given the strong association between psychopathy and recidivism in the adult literature (Harris, Rice, & Cormier, 1991; Rice & Harris, 2013; Swogger, Walsh, Christie, Priddy, & Conner, 2015), might we find similar associations among serious juvenile offenders with callous–unemotional traits?

In our opinion, the current literature indeed suggests that juvenile offenders with callous–unemotional traits are at an increased likelihood of reoffending (Asscher et al., 2011); however, there is strong evidence indicating that forensic evaluators should exercise caution when making predictions about the likelihood that youth with psychopathic traits will reoffend. For instance, a study by Cauffman, Kimonis, Dmitrieva, and Monahan (2009) used three different tools to assess for juvenile psychopathy, two of which had been validated in prior studies, the Psychopathy Checklist: Youth Version (PCL:YV) and the Youth Psychopathic Traits Inventory (YPI). A third measure, the NEO Psychopathy Resemblance Index, had never been used in a study to identify the presence of juvenile psychopathy. Among this study's sample comprised of 1,200 "serious male juvenile offenders" the correlations between juvenile psychopathy and the likelihood of reoffense, while noteworthy over the short-term, dropped significantly during a three-year period. Also, youth who met criteria for juvenile psychopathy on one rating scale often did not meet criteria for psychopathy on the others. The authors argue that

> given the PCL:YV's inability to predict long-term behavior, it would be ethically inappropriate to use such a measure to decide matters

such as whether a defendant should be tried as a juvenile or as an adult or whether an adolescent should be sentenced to a treatment facility or to life in prison without possibility of parole. (Cauffman et al., 2009, p. 13)

While we share the authors' ethical concerns, we would also caution readers not to get carried away in their condemnation of such tools. In our view, a thorough forensic evaluation of a juvenile offender might reasonably incorporate one or more of these or similar rating scales, so long are they are not the only means of determining the disposition of a minor. Later on in this chapter we discuss the use of structured risk assessment tools that rely on the most salient aspects of the violence risk literature in order to help guide forensic evaluations.

An additional reason for exercising caution in relying on the presence of psychopathic traits, which is essentially a genetic, physiologic, and characterologic propensity for cold aggression, to predict future violence and recidivism is the presence of evidence suggesting that some adolescents with psychopathic are amenable to treatment. A noteworthy study by Caldwell, Skeem, Salekin, and Van Rybroek (2006) involved 141 male juvenile offenders who scored highly on the PCL:YV. The boys who participated in this study were divided between "an intensive treatment program" versus "treatment as usual." The youth who received the treatment as usual condition were over two times more likely to have a violent reoffense during the course of a two-year follow-up period. We cite this study because it is a straightforward example of how a well-informed developmental psychopathology perspective is consistent with advancements in the juvenile psychopathy literature. In other words, we argue that this study is consistent with our viewpoint that developmental courses have the potential to change when some of the issues perpetuating maladaptive development are addressed.

In summary, the literature on juvenile desistance is overall reassuring. There is evidence suggesting that juvenile offenders with propensities for acts of cold aggression, otherwise known as callous–unemotional or psychopathic traits, carry a higher risk for violent recidivism. That said, our ability to predict the likelihood that a minor will violently reoffend based on the tools we have available to measure the presence of juvenile psychopathy alone is inadequate. Further complicating forensic psychiatrists' and psychologists' ability to make clear-cut decisions about the chances of redemption of juvenile offenders with psychopathic traits or, to put another way, their "amenability to treatment," is that their characters are not fully formed and there is evidence suggesting that they can, in some cases, respond to treatment.

6.6 Sociodemographic Factors

According to the Office of Juvenile Justice and Delinquency Prevention (2015), the overall rate of juvenile arrests in the United States has trended downward in recent years. That said, concern for disparities continue to exist along racial and socioeconomic lines, although the data regarding socioeconomic and racial disparities is somewhat mixed (Gillis & Bath, 2016; Piquero, 2008; Tapia, 2010; Vazsonyi & Chen, 2010). However, a troubling development over the past 20 years is the rapid increase in the proportion of girls that are entering the juvenile justice system (Levintova, 2015) For instance, female juvenile offenders accounted for only 20% of all juvenile arrests in 1992, and that figure rose to 29% by 2012 (Sherman & Balck, 2015).

Sherman and Balck (2015) point out that girls tend to be the victims of a paternalistic and overprotective system, causing them to be detained more readily than boys for minor offenses. In addition, the authors assert that the majority of crimes that girls are detained for are closely related to the aftermath of traumatic experiences that were never tended to. For example, girls in juvenile detention tend to be the victims of sexual assault at approximately 4.5 times the rate of boys. Racial and ethnic disparities are particularly noteworthy among girls in juvenile detention with the population of African American girls growing most rapidly. Another troubling finding from Sherman and Balck's (2015) work is that detained girls, especially Latinas, are significantly more likely to die by age 29. A study by Cauffman, Feldman, Watherman, and Steiner (1998) was one of the first to look at the prevalence of mental health problems among incarcerated girls. Cauffman and colleagues found that the rate of posttraumatic stress disorder (PTSD) among incarcerated girls was greater that of the general population and incarcerated boys. These data make it clear that our juvenile justice system needs to do a better job of adapting to the needs of the girls and young women it serves, particularly those who are members of ethnic minorities that have been marginalized in the United States both historically and in the present.

Vignette

Mary was a 14-year-old girl from Antioch, California, who lived with her mother, stepfather, and two older brothers. Mary had a history of academic difficulties, occasionally cut school, and smoked marijuana several times per week. Mary attended a party with some older girls she knew from her neighborhood. At the party were a group of older men that she did not know. At some point that evening Mary blacked out and woke up in a van surrounded by four adult men. Mary was kept in an abandoned house and repeatedly sexually assaulted over the course of one week until she was able to escape after being left alone, flag down a passing motorist, and ask for help. Mary experienced frequent nightmares and a variety of symptoms related to PTSD over the course of two months after returning home; however, she was not enrolled in any treatment and the men who kidnapped her had not been brought to justice. Mary visited a friend who was having a small get-together and noticed a teenage boy and girl she had been acquainted with in the past but did not know well making out on the couch. Mary became incensed and demanded that the couple take their behavior someplace else. An argument ensued between Mary and the other teenage girl. While the two girls were face to face, Mary picked up a glass from a nearby table and smashed it over the other girl's head. She then proceeded to kick her in the face and abdomen while she lay on the ground until other teens at the party were able to pull her off. The teenage girl that Mary hit sustained a concussion and several bruised ribs and required multiple stitches above her left eye. Mary was taken into custody and eventually released into the care of her parents. I was asked to perform Mary's trial competency evaluation. After reviewing the police report, collateral sources of information including school records and interviews with her parents, and meeting with Mary it became clear that she was suffering from severe PTSD. Mary's ongoing symptoms at the time of our meeting were notable for initial insomnia, frequent nightmares, intrusive memories, avoidance of being alone with men, and feeling constantly "on guard" with an inability to relax. Mary had also been argumentative with peers, teachers, and family alike and prone to crying spells since returning home. She reported feeling justified in assaulting the girl due to concerns for her safety and was unable to discuss the details of her case without shaking and breaking down. My report for the juvenile court stated that Mary needed to receive much-needed treatment for PTSD before adjudication.

The Northwestern Juvenile Project looked at psychiatric disorders among 1,829 youth in juvenile detention between the ages of 10 and 18. Approximately two-thirds of boys and 75% of girls in this study met criteria for one or more psychiatric disorders. When the diagnosis of conduct disorder was excluded, almost 60% of boys and over two-thirds of girls had impairments related to one or more psychiatric disorders. Approximately half of all detained boys and girls met criteria for a substance use disorder (Teplin et al., 2002; Teplin et al., 2013). While these figures are staggering, there is evidence suggesting that these data may underestimate the degree of psychopathology of detained youth, a significant portion of whom meet criteria for DBDs.

As part of the close collaboration between Stanford University's Division of Child and Adolescent Psychiatry and what was once called the CYA, a series of papers and a report was provided to then-Governor Gray Davis to examine the psychopathology among incarcerated youth. Overall, our findings were comparable with the previous findings by Teplin and colleagues in Chicago (2002, 2013) that are summarized earlier in this chapter. In fact, as Box 6.1 illustrates, a vast majority of the youth admitted to the CYA between August and December of 2001 who took part in our studies met diagnostic criteria for three or more mental disorders. The figure also illustrates how incarcerated girls tended to have a great deal more comorbid psychiatric illness than incarcerated boys. In essence, the juvenile justice system had become a refuge of last resort for poor and disenfranchised youth, many of whom have pressing mental health needs (Steiner et al., 2001).

A study by Karnik and colleagues (2010) examined the prevalence of psychiatric disorders among incarcerated nine months after incarceration according to ethnicity/race and age. The findings from this study included evidence that incarcerated boys and girls were most likely to meet criteria for DBD, older incarcerated boys were the most likely to have a substance use disorder, and minority youth overall reported less psychiatric symptoms, which meant that white youth in this study had the highest levels of psychopathology. Another salient finding from this study is that incarcerated youth who were nine months postadjudication reported higher rates of psychopathology than previous research by Teplin and colleagues (2002; Karnik et al., 2010). For example, 94% of the boys age 16 or younger and who were 17 years and older in this study met criteria for conduct disorder. Surprisingly, 97% of incarcerated girls age 16 and younger and 87% of girls age 17 or older met criteria for conduct disorder. In our view, there are multiple possible explanations for the higher rates of psychopathology among incarcerated youth postadjudication, particularly those with DBDs, which include the following hypotheses:

1. The sheer stress of juvenile incarceration may exacerbate underlying psychopathology among incarcerated youth.
2. Youth with higher levels of psychopathology may be more likely to commit offenses resulting in postadjudication incarceration.
3. Incarcerated youth with DBDs may have less incentive to minimize the extent of previous maladaptive and/or antisocial behaviors consistent with a DBD diagnosis after adjudication.

For instance, it stands to reason that the perceived risk of endorsing multiple symptoms associated with conduct disorder would be lower once the juvenile court has already made its decisions. One thing that is abundantly clear is that there is a startling number of DBDs among juvenile justice involved youth. This overlap is why we feel strongly about the importance of including a chapter on the forensic implications of DBDs for this text. Also, regardless of the reasons for the overall high rates of mental disorders among juvenile justice involved youth, particularly incarcerated youth, it is clear that ready access to quality psychiatric care among this population is essential.

6.7 The Elements of a Crime and Aggression Subtypes

Next we discuss the ramifications that juvenile offenders' personal tendencies toward acts of hot versus cold aggression may have on their disposition in juvenile or adult courts. First we cover the basic elements of all crime, that is, the *actus reus* (i.e., act forbidden by law) and *mens rea* (i.e., the guilty intent to commit said forbidden act). *Mens rea* is further subdivided into different levels, which can have major implications within criminal and juvenile courts. The levels of *mens rea* typically involved in criminal cases refer to whether acts were done in a manner that was purposeful (i.e., intending to engage in a criminal activity or cause a criminal result), performed knowingly (i.e., in a conscious manner with the intent of causing harm), reckless (i.e., knowingly taking a substantial and unjustifiable risk), or with negligence (i.e., unintentionally placing others in harms' way when one should have been able to recognize the risk to others).

Earlier in this chapter we briefly reviewed Ash's (2012) article on evaluating culpability in adolescents. In general, adolescents are not considered as fully responsible for antisocial acts as adults due to their developmental immaturity; however, the extent to which this is the case can vary a great deal. In the case of very serious alleged offenses (e.g., murder), juveniles in most jurisdictions can be transferred, or "waived," to adult court. The rules that mediate decisions on whether to transfer juveniles to adult court include both clear-cut "objective" criteria (i.e., age, charge, prior record) and somewhat vague and subjective "discretionary" criteria (e.g., a youth's "dangerousness" or "amenability to treatment") criteria (Fagan & Deschenes, 1990). Thus evidence indicating the level of *mens rea* involved in an alleged crime, a youth's pattern of antisocial acts, and/or perceived amenability to treatment may become significant considerations in some jurisdictions. For instance, has the juvenile in question displayed a pattern of repeated acts of cold predatory aggression, or is the pattern more consistent with explosive episodes of reactive aggression in response to perceived threat?

The term *diminished capacity* refers to instances in which a defendant lacked the capacity to form the necessary *mens rea* (i.e., guilty intent) that went along with an unlawful act due to mental disease or intoxication. We discuss two famous examples of a diminished capacity defense from adult criminal cases to illustrate what diminished capacity means. In the 1991 case of *People v. Saille* the defendant, Mr. Manuel De Jesus Saille, killed a patron, Ms. Guadalupe Borba, at a neighborhood bar. Mr. Sallie had been drinking all day prior to his arrival at a local tavern called Eva's Café. The security guard at Eva's Cafe, Mr. David Ballagh, refused to allow Mr. Saille entrance to Eva's Cafe on two separate occasions that night due to his drunken state. Mr. Saille threatened to kill Mr. Ballagh after he was rebuffed a second time and later returned to Eva's Café around 1 AM with a semiautomatic assault rifle. A struggle between Mr. Sallie and Mr. Ballagh ensued, resulting in Mr. Saille's assault rifle firing and killing Ms. Borba. Mr. Saille was charged with first-degree murder and sought to have his charge reduced to manslaughter because he was drunk when he killed Ms. Borba. A trial court, court of appeals, and the California Supreme Court all disagreed with Mr. Saille. The California Supreme Court ultimately ruled that voluntary intoxication alone was insufficient grounds to reduce Mr. Saille's crime from first-degree murder to a lesser charge of manslaughter.

Perhaps the most famous example of a diminished capacity defense comes from San Francisco Board of Supervisors member Dan White's trial for shooting and killing Mayor George Moscone and Supervisor Harvey Milk in 1978. Some readers may be familiar with the term "Twinkie Defense" coined by members of the media who covered this case even if they do not know the following details. A forensic psychologist from the San Francisco Bay Area, Dr. Martin Blinder, opined that Dan White's diet of Coca-Cola and Twinkies leading up to the murders of Mayor Moscone and Supervisor Milk likely exacerbated his already deeply depressed state, thereby resulting in a diminished capacity to formulate guilty intent (i.e., *mens rea*). In the case of juveniles, we can apply the concept of developmental immaturity as a means of a juvenile being less culpable, as the Chicago reformers mentioned at the outset of this book advocated.

6.8 Risk Assessment Tools

Vignette

Sebastian was six years old when he was molested by a male neighbor. He was 11 years old when he began smoking marijuana, and by age 13 he had been caught for shoplifting on three occasions. During high school,

Sebastian had a learning disorder with an individualized education plan. He had passing grades and was a backup offensive lineman on his high school football team. He liked girls but was far too shy to approach them on his own. When Sebastian was 16 he began secretly dating an 11-year-old girl in the seventh grade that he had met online. Their courtship seemed innocent at first; they sent messages on social media and occasionally held hands when they were alone. One evening, Sebastian asked to meet his young girlfriend after football practice. The two began to kiss and when the girl became overwhelmed, she told Sebastian, "I don't like you like that" and tried to back away; he would not let her go. He eventually punched her multiple times and sexually assaulted her. Sebastian told the girl not to tell anyone about what had happened. The girl developed PTSD and eventually confided to her friends about the incident. Sebastian was taken into custody, and the juvenile court requested sexual offender risk assessment prior to adjudication.

There are a variety of formal risk assessment tools that are used to assess youth violence and/or sexual violence risk. Some of these risk assessments are "actuarial" in nature meaning that they provide a percentage likelihood of reoffending within a given amount of time. Actuarial tools typically rely on historical or "static" risk factors (i.e., predictor variables that do not change over time) to estimate the probability of future violence and/or recidivism. One example of an actuarial juvenile violence risk assessment tool is the Youth Assessment and Screening Instrument (YASI). The YASI is designed for juvenile offenders between the ages of 12 and 18 and is typically scored by juvenile justice case workers. Another risk assessment tool that is based on an actuarial model is the Juvenile Sex Offender Assessment Protocol–II (J-SOAP-II). Although the J-SOAP-II is structured like an actuarial risk assessment tool, its developers did not have enough data from a large enough sample of juvenile sexual reoffenders to provide probabilities of reoffending. As a result, the J-SOAP-II is most accurately described as a structured professional judgment tool or, in the words of its creators, "an empirically informed guide for the systematic review and assessment of a uniform set of items that may reflect increased risk to reoffend" (Prentky & Righthand, 2003, p. 11).

Some risk assessments are based primarily on "structured" or "guided" clinical assessment, utilizing a checklist of factors that the extant professional literature has identified as important risk factors for violence (Borum, 2000). In other words, these tools ask evaluators to use their own professional judgments to rate the severity of risk factors that are empirically supported. These sorts of risk assessments are often aptly referred to as "structured professional judgment" tools. A structured professional judgment approach does not provide a percentage or odds of reoffending like actuarial tools. Instead, a structured professional judgment approach allows clinicians to make more individualized appraisals of a person's risk for violence and/or reoffending based on important considerations derived from the literature. In some scenarios, evaluators are able to combine both actuarial and structured professional judgment tools when performing a risk assessment. An example of a commonly used structured professional judgment tool used with juveniles is the Structured Assessment of Violence Risk for Youth (Borum, 2006).

We have referenced the topic of psychopathy and juvenile psychopathy throughout previous chapters. We next briefly discuss a tool that is used to assess for psychopathic traits in minors, the PCL:YV (Forth, Kosson, Hare, Sevecke, & Krischer, 2014). The PCL:YV is an adaptation of the Hare Psychopathy Checklist–Revised (PCL-R), a commonly used measure of psychopathy in adults (Hare & Vertommen, 1991). The adult version or PCL-R was originally developed as a research tool to measure the construct of psychopathy; however, its results tend to highly correlate with violent recidivism, making it a commonly used instrument in violence risk assessments.

The PCL-R and PCL:YV have been the subject of some controversy. For example, a study with 22 participants by Miller, Rufino, Boccaccini, Jackson, and Murrie (2011) found that the PCL-R scores provided by examiners varied based on the examiner's personality traits. In addition, there is evidence suggesting that some forensic experts performing violence risk assessments are more likely to score the PCL-R in accordance with the views of the side (i.e., prosecution versus defense) that retained them (Murrie, Boccaccini, Guarnera, & Rufino, 2013; Murrie et al., 2009). In regard to the construct of juvenile psychopathy and the PCL:YV, there is data suggesting that psychopathic traits among youth are reliable indicators of future recidivism indicating that the PCL:YV is an important tool for the early identification of youth at risk for psychopathy (Corrado, Vincent, Hart, & Cohen, 2004; Kosson, Cyterski, Steuerwald, Neumann, & Walker-Matthews, 2002; Lynam, Caspi, Moffitt, Loeber, & Stouthamer-Loeber, 2007). Additional data suggests that some measures of psychopathic traits in juveniles, including the PCL:YV, does a decent job of predicting future violent recidivism in boys (Schmidt et al, 2006) but lacks a high level of predictive validity for girls (Odgers, Reppucci, & Moretti, 2005; Schmidt, Campbell, & Houlding, 2011; Schmidt, McKinnon, Chattha, & Brownlee, 2006). A recent study looking at young Australian offenders concluded that the while PCL:YV was able to identify severely antisocial youth, it did not do a good job of distinguishing potentially psychopathic from nonpsychopathic youth (Shepherd & Strand, 2016). The same study found that neither the PCL:YV nor another well-known measure of juvenile psychopathy, the YPI, were able to identify recidivists from nonrecidivists. It is beyond the scope of this text to debate the merits of risk assessments commonly used on juvenile justice involved youth; however, we think it is important for clinicians who work with youth who have significant behavior problems to be aware of these instruments, their intended purpose, and some of the debate within our field that surrounds their use.

Before proceeding, we provide some background on the Weinberger Adjustment Inventory (WAI). The WAI consists of 84 questions designed to assess a person's social-emotional adjustment in response to stressors. The WAI asks subjects to rate their level of agreement with its questions on a scale of 1 through 5, with 1 meaning "false" and 5 meaning "true." The subscales of the WAI address a person's level of impulse control, ability to suppress aggression, empathy or "consideration of others," and "temperance," otherwise known as self-restraint (Feldman & Weinberger, 1994; Weinberger, Feldman, Ford, & Chastain, 1987; Weinberger & Schwartz, 1990). Figure 6.1 depicts the four adaptive stress styles characterized in the WAI, which are the Reactive (i.e., individuals who are report experiencing high distress and limited ability to restrain impulses), Suppressor (i.e., those who report experiencing high levels of distress along with the ability to control their impulses), Nonreactive (i.e., respondents who report low levels of distress in conjunction with limited impulse control), and Repressor (i.e., persons who self-report low levels of distress and high levels of impulse control in response to stress) types. Interestingly, the WAI has been shown to correlate well with perhaps the most famous and well-validated personality test in existence, the Minnesota Multiphasic Personality Inventory among incarcerated adolescent males (Huckaby, Kohler, Garner, & Steiner, 1998).

At this point some of the adaptive styles in the WAI sound a bit familiar. We have previously talked about how individuals with psychopathic traits are less prone to experience fear in response to threat and have a tendency to

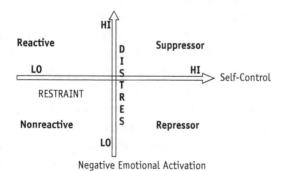

Figure 6.1 Weinberger Adjustment Inventory, adaptive style by distress and restraint.
Source: Weinberger & Schwartz (1990).

be impulsive when satisfying their desires. We have also discussed how individuals prone to reactive aggression tend to exhibit high levels of distress in response to perceived threat and lash out due to poor impulse control. In our opinion, the "Nonreactive" and "Reactive" adaptive styles characterized in the WAI map on fairly well to the cold versus hot aggression subtypes, respectively. In addition, a number of studies have shown a clear relationship between low levels of self-control and delinquency, which, as we will see, makes the WAI a particularly interesting and useful instrument (Cauffman, Steinberg, & Piquero, 2005; Fine, Steinberg, Frick, & Cauffman, 2016; Moffitt et al., 2011; Steinberg et al., 2008).

A study by Steiner, Cauffman, and Duxbury (1999) showed that the risk of recidivism among adolescent males can be predicted by personality traits observed on the WAI. In this study, the WAI was administered to 481 boys incarcerated in the CYA then followed 148 longitudinally for up to 4.5 years after their release from custody. This study found that nearly 90% of the boys whose profile on the WAI classified them as "Nonreactive," that is, those who reported low levels of distress (i.e., less negatively emotionally impacted by incarceration) and low levels of self-restraint (i.e., more prone to act aggressively in response to a variety of stressors), on the WAI were rearrested within 4.5 years following their release (Steiner et al., 1999). In contrast, a group labeled as "Suppressors," that is, those who reported feeling highly distressed during their incarceration in addition to reporting high levels of self-restraint, were the least likely group to be arrested within the same time period at a rate of around 44%. In addition, 71% of the Reactive subgroup and 62% of the boys in the Repressor group were arrested within 4.5 years after release. This study is important because it is one of the first studies to show how adaptive styles can be used as a means of predicting risk of reoffense among youth.

A more recent example of the utility of the adaptive styles assessed by the WAI in risk assessment is observed in a study by Fine and colleagues (2016). This asked the question of whether a self-report measure like the WAI, behaviors observed in a laboratory, or some combination thereof were best for predicting the likelihood of adolescent reoffending. This study involved 930 teenage boys between the ages of 13 and 17 who completed the WAI and participated in a laboratory based Go/NoGo response inhibition task. The Go/NoGo task required participants to look at a computer screen and push the associated keyboard's space bar every time a solitary letter briefly appeared on the screen; however, participants were instructed not to press the space bar every time they were shown the letter X. The letter X only appeared one-quarter of the time, making it more likely that participants would not inhibit their response whenever the less frequently appearing Xs showed up on the screen. Participants who were more likely to press the space bar whenever the X appeared (i.e., those who were more likely to produce "commission errors") were deemed as having lesser degrees of impulse control. This study showed that a self-report measure (i.e., the WAI) was superior to the laboratory test of impulse control in predicting the likelihood of reoffending over both the short and long term. In fact, the laboratory-based Go/NoGo task did not offer any additional information that was helpful for predicting recidivism when used in conjunction with the WAI. This study is important because it is the first to demonstrate that self-report measures like the WAI, which includes items that are applicable to the real-world experiences of youth (e.g., "I should try harder to control myself when I'm having fun" or "People who get me angry better watch out"), are superior to laboratory tasks that are devoid of context when assessing violence risk. From our perspective, the studies mentioned previously are further evidence that the developmental perspective on psychopathology espoused in this book is based on a solid theoretical framework and empiricism, as opposed to some of the taxonomy and nomenclature within the *Diagnostic and Statistical Manual of Mental Disorder* (DSM).

Vignettte, Continued

Not long after Sebastian was taken into custody, a younger male cousin revealed that he had been molested by him on several occasions. While Sebastian was upset about everything that had occurred leading up to his arrest, he had a tough time relating an appreciation for the gravity of his actions or the distress he had caused the other children involved. Although Sebastian's risk assessment revealed some protective factors including positive relationships with football coaches and teammates and adapting well to his new surroundings in custody, becoming a model of good behavior for the other boys, he was deemed to be a moderate to high overall risk to the community and in need of a comprehensive treatment that included multisystemic therapy following his release from juvenile detention.

6.9 Outpatient Treatment Approaches for Juvenile Justice Involved Youth

Multisystemic Therapy (MST) is a cost-effective family and community-based approach designed to treat youth who are entrenched in the juvenile justice system, are dealing with serious emotional disturbances, and/or have accompanying substance use problems (Henggeler & Sheidow, 2012; Klietz, Borduin, & Schaeffer, 2010; Schoenwald, Ward, Henggeler, Pickrel, & Patel, 1996; Sheidow et al., 2004). The reported cost-effectiveness of MST becomes even more salient when one considers findings from McCollister, French, and Fang (2010) that provides per unit cost estimates based on court fees, police investigations, cost of incarceration, and so on for a variety of crimes ranging from murder (e.g., approximately $9 million per murder) to stolen property (e.g., approximately $8,000 per stolen property offense). At its core, MST seeks to address the environmental factors that perpetuate conduct problems, juvenile delinquency, and substance abuse. MST therapists work with families by going into their homes, establishing stronger relationships their child's school (e.g., involving teachers and school administrators), and recruiting help from available community resources (e.g., connecting families with positive local resources and role models). MST therapists seek to accomplish their goals through a collaborate problem-solving approach and being on call for a family 24 hours per day over the course of treatment, which can last anywhere from three to five months. MST therapists help caretakers progressively increase the level of monitoring for their child and address disciplinary concerns on their own throughout the course of treatment. The therapist's goal is not to become a fixture a family's life but rather to help the family learn to function better on their own.

MST has its roots in a variety of theoretical models. For example, Urie Bronfenbrenner's (1979) ecological system's theory asserts that youth grow up within multiple systems (e.g., family, neighborhood, school, peer groups) that influence their behaviors and developmental trajectories. Some of these systems directly impact behaviors (e.g., parenting styles), while others exert their influence on youth in more indirect ways (e.g., the negative effects that a lack of needed social services has on a family). The MST model applies Bronfenbrenner's ideas on child development to antisocial behaviors in youth. In other words, if we want to effectively address conduct problems, we need to first take into account the variety of systems that are exerting an influence on youth and their behaviors (Henggeler & Sheidow, 2012). Additional influences on MST's development include Salvador Minuchin's model for structural family therapy, Jay Haley's model for strategic therapy, Albert Bandura's social learning theory, and the problem-solving approach emphasized in cognitive behavioral therapy (Henggeler & Sheidow, 2012). Multiple studies, some of which we discuss later, have shown MST to have benefits that include reductions in recidivism, less substance abuse, improved family functioning, and a decreased likelihood that the younger siblings of youth who receive MST will develop similar problems of their own (Henggeler, 2012; Henggeler, Melton, & Smith, 1992; van der Stouwe, Asscher, Stams, Deković, & van der Laan, 2014; Wagner, Borduin, Sawyer, & Dopp, 2014).

A randomized controlled trial performed by Butler, Baruch, Hickey, and Fonagy (2011) in the United Kingdom looked at the effectiveness of MST in reducing juvenile offenses and the need for removal of youth from their homes versus treatment as usual in a large ethnically diverse urban population. This study is important because, relative to the United States, the United Kingdom had more robust support services available for juvenile offenders when this experiment took place. For instance, the services available in the UK around this time included Youth Offender Teams whose purpose was to prevent juvenile offenses. This study set out to address concerns that MST's reported "effectiveness" was primarily due to the absence of coordinated efforts in the United States to meet the needs of juvenile delinquent populations. In other words, is the theoretical framework and fidelity implementation (i.e., the delivery of MST in the manner it was designed to be implemented) of MST particularly well suited to its target population, or is it simply better than nothing?

Butler and colleagues (2011) concluded that both MST and treatment as usual (i.e., reliance on Youth Offender Teams) led to reductions in offending; however, the fidelity implementation of MST led to marked reductions in nonviolent reoffending 18 months posttreatment as compared to treatment as usual. Parental reports of aggressive and delinquent behavior and participants self-report of delinquency were also markedly reduced in the MST population relative to treatment as usual. This study indicates that MST can be a highly effective tool when it is applied using rigorous quality control standards and adds value to communities' existing programs to address the needs of juvenile justice involved youth.

Another international study in 2011 by Rhiner, Graf, Dammann, and Fuerstenau looked at the implementation of MST in Switzerland with 70 teenagers and their families. While not an randomized controlled trial, this study showed that youth whose families participated in MST had improved overall levels of functioning psychosocial functioning at the conclusion of treatment. In addition, at six-month follow-up over 90% of youth who completed MST were still living in their family's home, had remained in school or vocational training, and had not committed new "chargeable offenses." At 18-month follow-up the previously mentioned success measures were maintained at a rate of 80% or better in all three categories. This study is further evidence of MST's effectiveness across cultures and how its impact extends beyond that of mere "symptom control" and addresses some of the root causes of conduct problems such as a lack of parental/caregiver agency, fosters continued access to education or job training, and avoids the self-perpetuating cycle of juvenile justice system involvement (Rhiner et al., 2011).

For readers who are still wondering if MST is the "real deal" based on the studies we have referenced, we would like to re-direct attention to the meta-analysis we referenced in Chapter 5 by van der Stouwe and colleagues (2014) examining MST's effectiveness. MST was shown to have a number of benefits that included reductions in juvenile delinquency, out of home placements, and substance use. As we conclude our discussion of MST, it bears repeating that adherence to the protocol set forth by MST's developers is associated with better outcomes (Henggeler, 2012), thus providing a rationale for the high level of training and fidelity monitoring required by the organization responsible for accrediting MST programs, MST Services.

A meta-analysis by Baldwin, Christian, Berkeljon, and Shadish (2012) compared Brief Stragegic Family Therapy, Functional Family Therapy, Multidimensional Family Therapy, and MST in the treatment of teen substance abuse and reduction of juvenile delinquency. All of the interventions were compared to a control group, some alternate form of therapy, or treatment as usual. This meta-analysis found that all four of the approaches were only somewhat more effective than treatment as usual or alternate approaches. That said, this meta-analysis was underpowered (i.e., too small a sample size to detect meaningful differences between groups) and no conclusions could be drawn when comparing one of the four approaches versus the other or control groups. This meta-analysis reflects the paucity of research on effective treatments for conduct problems. It also indicates that approaches to targeting antisocial behavior in youth that are based on a developmentally sound theoretical framework are more effective than ad hoc alternatives.

A small study (Shelton et al., 2011) looked at the efficacy of a 16-week dialectical behavioral therapy program that had been modified for use in correctional settings with incarcerated males between the ages of 16 and 19. There were some limitations with this study, including small sample size (e.g., only 26 of the original 38 participants completed the trial), the absence of a control group, and a lack of data on participants' behavior after the treatment program was completed. Despite these significant limitations, there were some promising findings that included reductions in participants' levels of physical aggression and fewer disciplinary infractions while in custody.

While the findings of this paper are encouraging, we have additional concerns that were not addressed by the authors due to the absence of information on the participants' preexisting mental health diagnoses, if any. A particular concern we have about the lack of data regarding psychiatric histories is due to the fact that most youth in correctional settings have conduct problems. Dialectical Behavior Therapy is a treatment modality that relies heavily on a group therapy component. A great deal of research supports the notion that engaging in group therapy where a significant portion of the participants have conduct disorder and/or have active substance use problems is counterproductive and may actually exacerbate problem behaviors (Dishion, McCord, & Poulin, 1999; Santisteban et al., 2003; Szapocznik & Prado, 2007). However, the information provided in this study did not indicate whether participants had a preincarceration diagnosis of conduct disorder and/or whether they continued to meet criteria for conduct disorder. In general, we advise caution when it comes to referring youth with conduct disorder to group therapy as there is some evidence suggesting the extant literature and personal experience indicates that these youth tend to "find each other," positively reinforce negative behavior among themselves (e.g., some have referred to this process as "deviancy training"), and may effectively commandeer the group (e.g., Arnold & Hughes, 1999; De Haan & MacDermid, 1999; Dishion et al., 1999; Fo & O'Donnell, 1975). That said, more recent meta-analyses have suggested that the evidence suggesting that treating delinquent and/or youth with conduct disorders in group therapy is counterproductive is be a bit overblown (Lipsey, 2006; Weiss et al., 2005). The decision on whether or not to treat youth with conduct disorders in group settings has significant implications given that the implementation of group therapies tend to be less costly and have the potential of reaching many more youth.

6.10 Clinical Implications

Treating juvenile justice involved youth is complex task that involves the coordination of multiple providers and systems of care, which include the juvenile court, juvenile probation services, forensic evaluators, county mental health providers, and case managers. In many cases, counties contract with outside agencies for the delivery of mental health care, thus adding another layer of complexity. Detained youth will also work with medical providers (e.g., primary care doctors, nurses, etc.), educational staff (e.g., teachers, paraprofessionals), and correctional officers who, in addition to being the eyes and ears of juvenile hall, often serve as the first points of contact during psychiatric emergencies.

Treating incarcerated youth offers some unique challenges that can include the systematic monitoring of violence and suicide risk. Additionally, the types of treatment offered in correctional settings are often different from what is available in the community. For instance, it is commonplace in correctional institutions, both adult and juvenile, to avoid prescribing medications that have the potential for abuse or carry a high "street value" or are highly sought after by those in detention. Some examples include benzodiazepines, stimulant medications, the antidepressant medication bupropion, the atypical antipsychotic medication quetiapine, and opiate pain relievers. Also, the availability of group and/or individual psychotherapy and substance abuse treatment, much like the budgets for such services, often varies from one county to another. Due to the high rates of psychiatric comorbidities among juvenile justice involved youth, treatment for this population should be multimodal and tailored to a youth's individual needs. We believe that child and adolescent psychiatrists are particularly well qualified to support and lead treatment teams (Steiner & Cauffman, 1998). In addition, pediatricians with a strong background in developmental approaches to understanding psychopathology (e.g., developmental behavioral pediatricians, pediatric addiction medicine specialists) have skill sets that are well suited for helping oversee the delivery of medical and psychiatric care to juvenile justice involved and incarcerated youth (Braverman & Murray, 2011). Child and adolescent psychiatrists and doctors from the mentioned pediatric subspecialties have a diverse skill set ranging from an understanding of psychopathology and appropriate psychosocial treatment interventions to experience prescribing and monitoring the use of medications, many of which can lead to medical comorbidities (e.g., individuals on lithium need to have their kidney and thyroid function closely monitored). In addition, the mentioned medical providers generally have experience interfacing with colleagues from related fields (e.g., child psychologists, social workers, case managers, teachers, parents, etc.) to ensure the continuity of care between hospital or institutional settings and the community.

6.10.1 A MODEL OF CARE OF YOUTH IN JUVENILE DETENTION

As pointed out earlier in this chapter, multiple mental health diagnoses tend to be the norm among those in juvenile detention. Given this heterogeneity, clinicians who provide care in this setting are often faced with the most complex cases in adolescent psychiatry. In addition, the psychiatrists who work in juvenile justice settings are typically not in control of this challenging and complex system. Further complicating this scenario is the fact that correctional officers have the formidable responsibility of looking after the well-being of detainees, juvenile hall staff, and themselves.

In order to illustrate our point that psychiatrists' duty to do no harm and act in the best interests of their patients at times conflicts with the needs of correctional institutions to keep everyone safe, we offer the following hypothetical scenario based our clinical experiences.

Vignette

Jay was a 16-year-old boy with a history of conduct disorder, metham-phetamine use disorder, and bipolar disorder who was being housed in juvenile detention after being charged with grand theft of an automobile. Jay had reportedly been abusing methamphetamine and minimally com-plaint with his regular medication, lithium, during the weeks leading up to his arrest. The psychiatrist at Jay's juvenile facility was a part-time consult-ant who rounded on patients once per week and resumed Jay's outpatient does of lithium. Three days into Jay's stay at juvenile hall he refused to have his lithium level drawn and it became clear that he'd been "cheeking" (i.e., spitting out) his medication. Jay had also trashed his cell, punched a peer with whom he'd previously had some degree of "bad blood" outside of custody during dinner, and kicked the correctional officer who attempted to break up their skirmish in the knee, causing significant injury. Jay was ultimately placed in administrative segregation and had earned two assault charges by the time the consulting psychiatrist arrived to check in on him almost a week later. Correctional staff were aware of Jay's psychiatric his-tory; however, they attributed his assaultive behavior to negative attitudes and poor decision-making, rather than being emblematic of untreated mental illness. Jay was immediately transferred to an inpatient psychiatric facility after the psychiatrist met with him the following week.

Jay's story is all too common in modern health care. In the scenario described, physicians are given the ultimate responsibility for attending to a patient's well-being and mental health needs despite having limited decision-making powers. The situation involving Jay is a prime example of the ways that correctional staff charged with the monumental responsibility of ensuring the physical safety of all parties in these settings and treatment providers sometimes utilize conflict-ing approaches despite having similar goals. It is beyond the scope of this text to discuss trends in health-care policy; however, we outline what we believe is a common-sense approach to mental health care in juvenile detention, one with multiple clinical arms that cluster youth into groups based on their clinical histories and presentations as a means of more reliably addressing their mental health needs.

6.10.2 WHERE DO WE BEGIN?

We assert that the relationships between mental health treatment and psychiat-ric diagnoses are often less firm than they should be in juvenile detention, given the advancements in our understanding of best treatment practices. In our view, the previous statement is particularly evident in the use of medications for treating mental disorders and how institutions align or group youth in the system. The origins of this misalignment are complex and based, at least in part, on the following factors identified in the clinical and treatment needs assessment study for the CYA mentioned earlier in this chapter:

1. *Current nomenclature blurs lines between criminological and medical/psychological interventions and creates the impression that they are interchangeable.* At the same time, the system has clearly switched into a safety-first mode, which is applied indiscriminately across all individuals and all locations. Such an emphasis is not always justified, and there will be some cases where mental health treatment needs will dictate management within the institutions.
2. *The existing mental health system is fragmented, not unified.* It does not offer career trajectories to its practitioners. It deselects competent and energetic individuals by nature of the marginal compensation and isolation in the system.
3. *Lack of resources creates holes in service structure problems.*
4. *Isolation of mental health practitioners in the system from the management teams (school, criminological) deprives them of invaluable input to be received and output to give back to the team.*
5. *Education and training of mental health practitioners in the system is limited and thus, in combination with isolation, leads to idiosyncratic and outdated practices.*
6. *Youthful Offender Parole Board demands on the system are random and create pressures and demands that interfere with appropriate care.*

As was the case with the Youth Offender Parole Board, many counties see physicians and consultants, which means that juvenile detention facilities operate under a criminological model rather than a medical model based on developmental considerations. The information obtained on screening, clinical diagnoses, treatment plans, assignment to special programs, and continuity of care are often uneven between institutions despite the fact that most of them serve a similar population. Furthermore, the number of available beds, access to special programs designed for youth in custody, and the levels of expertise of the individuals running these programs vary in quality and are in need of more rigorous education and supervisory efforts. We see the rearrangement of mental health team components, a more centralized role for mental health providers in the management of detained youth, and the sophisticated coordination of the multilevel interventions required in juvenile detention as a means of addressing some of the shortcomings in how care is provided to those in juvenile detention.

6.10.3 WHAT DATA DO WE NEED, AND HOW CAN WE BEST SUMMARIZE THEM?

In this section we put forth a schematic of how juvenile detention facilities can cluster youth according to diagnoses in an efficient and effective manner. Our schematic is based largely on a report submitted to one-time California Governor Gray Davis that was funded by the NIJ and carried out in close partnership with the CYA (Steiner et al., 2001). Governor Gray Davis requested recommendations on how to best overhaul the way care is provided in juvenile detention. Although the study was carried out in 2001, we outline aspects that have continued relevance despite the passage of time. Also, to the best of our knowledge, there is not comparable data addressing adjudicated youth serving long-term sentences in juvenile detention facilities.

Before testing out ideas on how to improve the delivery of mental health care in juvenile detention, an exploratory data analysis was performed in order to generate clusters of psychiatric diagnoses that would yield meaningful results. Individual detained youth were clustered according to diagnostic information gained from the Structured Clinical Interview for DSM-IV Axis I Disorders (SCID-I) and the Structured Interview for DSM-IV Personality (SIDP-IV). These date were subjected to binary categorical cluster analyses to determine which diagnoses might cluster together and potentially streamline service delivery in a complex setting with frequently limited resources, like juvenile detention. The results of this cluster analysis are presented in Box 6.2 and Figure 6.2.

The statistical analyses produced five independent clusters: The first cluster that emerged, *Cluster I* (aka the "Emotion Disorder Cluster") consisted of mood disorders, anxiety disorders, borderline personality disorder, and oppositional defiant disorder. The fact that these disorders go together makes clinical sense, based on what we know of their etiology. They would primarily be treated with antidepressants, anti-anxiety agents, selective serotonin reuptake inhibitors, and mood stabilizers. Fifty percent of the youth who took part in our survey were present in this cluster.

Cluster II (aka the "Cognitive Cluster") consisted of detained youth with histories of psychosis, ADHD, and schizoid and schizotypal personality disorders. Fifteen percent of the youth involved in our analysis were present in this cluster. While there is some commonality of treatment across these diagnoses (e.g., antipsychotics, especially newer atypical antipsychotics), ADHD would be treated with stimulant medication, educational approaches specifically designed to target problems related to ADHD, behavior modification, and, nowadays, possibly even neurofeedback. Nevertheless, we believe these diagnoses can be thought of as a package because in contrast to Cluster I, where

---

Box 6.2 The Stanford/NIJ/CYA Project, 2001

CLUSTERING OF STRUCTURED SCID INTERVIEW DIAGNOSES

Cluster I: Mood, anxiety, borderline personality and oppositional defiant disorders, 50%

Cluster II: Psychosis, attention deficit hyperactivity, schizoid, and schizotypal disorders, 15%

Cluster III: Eating, somatoform, and adjustment disorders, 5%

Cluster IV: Alcohol and substance abuse (who do not fall into Clusters I–III), 20%

Cluster V: Alcohol and substance dependence (who do not fall into Clusters I–III), 27%

---

we find predominant disturbance of mood and affect, we would see predominant disturbance of cognition, thought, and attention (i.e., neuropsychiatric syndromes) in this grouping.

Cluster III consisted of disorders rarely seen in detained youth, and the comparisons to the frequencies in other populations reflect this fact. In contrast to Clusters I and II, disorders in this cluster tended to be coincidental. In our view, the diagnoses in this cluster probably do not reflect a special association to delinquent behavior, unlike the first two clusters. Specifically, Cluster III is comprised of eating disorders, somatoform disorders, and adjustment disorders. Of the

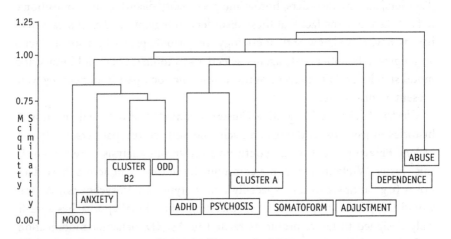

Figure 6.2 Cluster patterns of DSM-IV diagnoses by SCID interviews in incarcerated delinquents.

detained youth interviewed only 1% met the criteria for eating disorder, 2% for a somatoform disorder, and 3% for an adjustment disorder. Only 5% of the youth who participated in our survey were included in Cluster III. In addition to their rarity, these disorders also shared common methods of intervention: most likely we would track progress during incarceration (e.g., weight tracking), expecting improvement over time without any specific further intervention. A particularly useful tracking mechanism would be the visits to nurse or pediatrician tracking growth, nutritional status, and so on. Despite the fact that eating and somatoform disorders are more likely to be persistent, ultimately requiring treatment, adjustment disorders are usually transient, and maintaining a watchful eye on the ward with adjustment problems is the best treatment available.

Finally, the fourth and fifth clusters are comprised of substance use disorders. The DSM-5 no longer distinguishes from substance abuse (Cluster IV) versus substance dependence (Cluster V). Instead, substance use disorders are described on a continuum ranging from mild to moderate and severe. Classifying adolescents' issues with substance use along a continuum, whether it is the mild–moderate–severe distinction in the latest issue of the DSM or, as Stanford psychiatrist Dr. Anna Lembke has described, along a continuum of experimentation–limited use–problematic use, makes sense from a developmental psychopathology perspective (Steiner & Hall, 2015). The continuum of severity described in the DSM-5 seems especially appropriate when one considers the fact that scientific studies have never supported the idea that substance abuse was a precursor for substance dependence (Lembke, 2013). Such a continuum is also consistent with the ways they have been characterized in the literature, most notably in pediatrics, for years (Newcomb & Bentler, 1989; Shrier, Harris, Kurland, & Knight, 2003; Wilson, Sherritt, Gates, & Knight, 2004). One could think of Cluster IV as mild to moderate and Cluster V as severe in the DSM-5 terminology. This division has some important implications for treatment.

All these clustering analyses were conducted without the inclusion of DBDs, because they were present in almost all the subjects. Furthermore, only people who are not included in Cluster I through III are present in these two substance use clusters. That is, if a ward of the state met the criteria for depression and a severe cannabis use disorder, he would receive a score of "yes" for Cluster I but a score of "no" for Cluster IV. Cluster IV and Cluster V are mutually exclusive. Forty-seven percent of the subjects received a diagnosis relevant to substance use without a diagnosis present in one of the three other clusters. More specifically, 20% of the sample had milder substance use problems (i.e., met DSM-IV-TR criteria for substance abuse) and 27% had more severe problems (i.e., met DSM-IV-TR criteria for substance dependence), requiring long-term treatment.

Because rates of substance abuse and dependence, now under the umbrella of substance use disorders, were so high, the overlapping comorbidity with other mental health problems needed to be separated. Our expectation would be that juveniles who suffer from combinations of other disorders and substance use disorders would hopefully respond to intervention targeting their other comorbidities (e.g., depression). While mood problems can also arise from substance use, at this point we cannot confidently distinguish the order of events in this study. Future studies should focus on these developmental sequences.

6.10.4 THE IMPLICATIONS OF THESE FINDINGS FOR THE CREATION OF JUVENILE JUSTICE BASED FORENSIC PSYCHIATRY SERVICES

Despite the fact that our knowledge base is by no means complete, we are able to distill several salient treatment principles that have promise for success (Steiner, 1997). The nature and degree of psychopathology that associates with delinquency calls for several program characteristics that need to be implemented to increase our chances of success.

1. *Aiming for continua of care.* We expect that ultimately, a continuum of care model will provide the best vehicle for delivering state-of-the-art interventions. While morbidity is high, we expect that *extensive rather than intensive intervention* will be the basic model to address most of these problems. Finally, we expect that most children will require multimodal, carefully coordinated intervention, targeting multiple deficient domains. The main principle governing treatment will be that the ward be allowed to function in the least possible restrictive environment that is capable of ensuring safety and personal growth.
2. *Because juvenile delinquents are a highly heterogeneous group, with differing needs and levels of accompanying psychopathology, it is unrealistic to expect that any one intervention or even any one program will be equally effective for all members of such a diverse population.*
3. *There is little room for complacency or therapeutic nihilism.* The general message of recent investigations of program efficacy has been most succinctly stated by Loeber and Farrington (1998) in a summary of the accumulated wisdom of an expert panel on the issue: It is never too early and it is never too late.
4. *Multiple treatment targets should be selected,* as most of these youths are deficient in many domains of functioning.
5. *Most experts agree that there is little chance that isolated single interventions will be effective* against all forms of delinquency. Interventions need to be

multimodal; they need to be applied over sufficient lengths of time (i.e., over the course of months, not weeks). As much as is possible, they need to be delivered in settings that retain children in their social context to which they will return.

6. *Simple inoculation approaches and interventions based on single-event hypotheses are not going to be successful.*
7. *Services within the CYA need to reflect these principles.* Services should effectively combine criminological management and psychosocial and psychopharmacological interventions.

6.10.4.1 Specific Recommendations regarding Treatment Requirements with Juvenile Justice Populations

As a general principle, we suggest that the juvenile detention facilities would be best advised to treat the most prevalent problems that have evidence-based, tested treatments available and that have a very high chance of producing positive outcomes in terms of mental health as well as criminal recidivism. Diagnoses in Clusters I, II, and V would fulfill these criteria. There are special safety concerns that make Cluster II diagnoses somewhat more difficult to tackle. Programs and staffing should reflect the needs of wards with these diagnoses. We recognize that many difficult problems occur in this population, but some of them are infrequent, even rare, albeit extremely troublesome. Such problems should be probably handled by contracted arrangements. We think that such contracted arrangements can and should be made with other state entities, such as the Department of Mental Health. To saddle the juvenile correctional system with the care of the indigent underidentified, underserved, and undertreated mentally ill is tantamount to the criminalization of the mentally ill and not advised.

6.10.4.2 A Change in Vision: Creating a Coordinated Continuum of Criminological and Mental Health Interventions

Currently, the mental health services across the CYA and most likely many other juvenile justice facilities are characterized at best as adjunctive to juvenile justice and criminological rehabilitation and management and at worst as isolated and even irrelevant. The model is much like a solar system where a star (Juvenile Justice) is encircled by a very diverse array of planets (see Figure 6.3).

We suggest that on the basis of our findings, we need *to change this basic alignment to reflect more accurately the existing medical needs in this population.* Mental health services need to be an integral part of the ongoing criminological management of these wards. Depending on the severity and pervasiveness of disorders, mental health needs to play an increasingly prominent role with certain

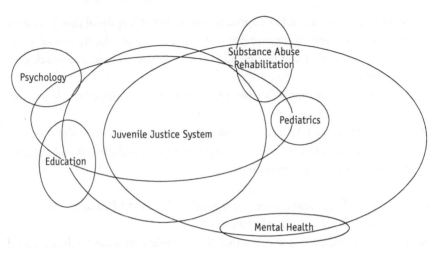

Figure 6.3 The solar system model of the relationship between juvenile justice and mental health systems in the California Youth Authority, 2001.

wards to the point of becoming the controlling influence in the management if severity or extensiveness of disorder warrants this.

To this end, we propose the following: We recommend that the psychiatric care for youth in general population be tantamount to intensive outpatient care provided nondetained youth in the community. In addition we recommend that special counseling programs be considered day treatment and that intensive treatment programs provide care similar to intensive inpatient or residential treatment facilities for nondetained youth, similar to the level of care associated with locked psychiatric inpatient units. Staffing at these facilities should be uniform across campuses with institutions being informed by best practices. The treatment settings we have described should be distributed in as geographically even a manner as possible across the state so that youth receiving treatment can be as close as possible to their communities and families as possible. Ensuring that youth are kept in close proximity to their communities will help facilitate continuity of care, preparatory programs, and family contact prior to discharge. We also recommend the establishment of institutions that specialize in treating certain diagnostic clusters in order to facilitate the more expert delivery of targeted services, staff development, and maximal recovery of the youth being cared for. It our recommendation that settings be created that can handle youth who are not overtly psychiatrically impaired yet present severe management problems (e.g., youth with strong histories of gang-related and/or predatory violence). These settings should be separate from the treatment settings described and utilize a criminologically informed management approach. We recommend that for this subset of youth, mental health only be provided on a consultation basis in order to best ensure the

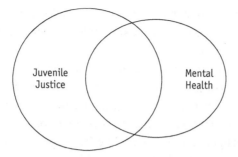

Figure 6.4 The integrated model of juvenile justice and mental health (Steiner et al., 2002).

safety of youth, correctional staff, and their care providers. The implementation of these recommendations would lead to an integrated model along the
lines of what we have illustrated in Figure 6.4 and discussed in great detail in
our report to Governor Davis.

Juvenile justice and mental health overlap to a considerable, although incomplete, degree. Juvenile justice and its interventions form the basis and backbone
of the needed services for these youths. Under ideal conditions, the system provides the necessary limits and boundaries of personal freedom, while appeal-
ing to personal responsibility. Mental health services should provide the care
necessary to restore youths to a level of functioning where they will maximally
benefit from juvenile justice interventions. At all times there must be a mutual
commitment to examine conjointly the most prudent and effective pathway to
intervene in a given case. Periodically, such a plan for intervention should be
examined and updated in the light of new information regarding the progress
of the youth.

6.11 Ethical Considerations

Early on in this chapter we talked about the US Supreme Court's recent decision
in the case of *Montgomery v. Louisiana*. The court's ruling made its decision in
the case of *Miller v. Alabama* retroactive, making it unconstitutional to sentence
someone who committed a murder while still a minor to life without the possibility of parole. An important caveat to the *Montgomery* ruling is that minors
who are deemed by the court to be "irreparably corrupt" or "permanently
incorrigible" may receive mandatory sentences of life without the possibility of
parole. This ruling raises some important questions for our courts to address
and, in our view, an ethical dilemma for forensic evaluators. For instance, recent
evidence suggests that the personalities of individuals continue to evolve and do
not plateau until around age 30 (Costa & McCrae, 1988; Terracciano, McCrae,

& Costa, 2010). How solid of a foundation does a forensic evaluator rely upon if he or she opines that a youth is not amenable to treatment and essentially has no hope for redemption?

Given the information presented in this text about our burgeoning understanding of psychopathy, evidence that some youth with callous–unemotional traits respond favorably to treatment, questions regarding the predictive validity of our risk assessments regarding the persistence of psychopathic traits into adulthood, and insights gathered from the Pathways to Desistance Study, can mental health professionals ethically opine with a degree of reasonable certainty that a minor is "irrepealably corrupt?" While the purpose of this book is not to answer this question, the *Montgomery* case provides an important example of the ways that legal philosophy and our ever-increasing understanding of the human condition do not always fit together neatly. It is our hope that this book will help further the discussion of how we can view our most at-risk youth, including those who commit violent crimes, in a developmentally sound and humanistic manner.

References

Alesina, A., & La Ferrara, E. (2014). A test of racial bias in capital sentencing. *The American Economic Review, 104*(11), 3397–3433.

American Academy of Psychiatry and the Law. (2014). About AAPL. http://www.aapl.org/org.htm

Arnold, M. E., & Hughes, J. N. (1999). First do no harm: Adverse effects of grouping deviant youth for skills training. *Journal of School Psychology, 37*(1), 99–115.

Ash, P. (2012). But he knew it was wrong: Evaluating adolescent culpability. *Journal of the American Academy of Psychiatry and the Law Online, 40*(1), 21–32.

Asscher, J. J., van Vugt, E. S., Stams, G. J. J., Deković, M., Eichelsheim, V. I., & Yousfi, S. (2011). The relationship between juvenile psychopathic traits, delinquency and (violent) recidivism: A meta-analysis. *Journal of Child Psychology and Psychiatry, 52*(11), 1134–1143.

Baldwin, S. A., Christian, S., Berkeljon, A., & Shadish, W. R. (2012). The effects of family therapies for adolescent delinquency and substance abuse: A meta-analysis. *Journal of Marital and Family Therapy, 38*(1), 281–304.

Bauer, S. M., Steiner, H., Feucht, M., Stompe, T., Karnik, N., Kasper, S., & Plattner, B. (2011). Psychosocial background in incarcerated adolescents from Austria, Turkey and former Yugoslavia. *Psychiatry Research, 185*(1), 193–199.

Borum, R. (2000). Assessing violence risk among youth. *Journal of clinical psychology, 56*(10), 1263–1288.

Borum, R. (2006). *Manual for the structured assessment of violence risk in youth (SAVRY).* Tampa: University of South Florida.

Braverman, P. K., & Murray, P. J. (2011). Health care for youth in the juvenile justice system. *Pediatrics, 128*(6), 1219–1235.

Bright, S. B. (1994). Counsel for the poor: The death sentence not for the worst crime but for the worst lawyer. *The Yale Law Journal, 103*(7), 1835–1883.

Bright, S. B. (2008). The Failure to Achieve Fairness: Race and Poverty Continue to Influence Who Dies. *U. Pa. J. Const. L., 11*, 23. (pages 1–16 – PDF online)

Bright, S. B. (2014). The role of race, poverty, intellectual disability, and mental illness in the decline of the death penalty. *University of Richmond Law Review, 49,* 671–692.

Bronfenbrenner, U. (1979). Contexts of child rearing: Problems and prospects. *American Psychologist, 34*(10), 844–850.

Butler, S., Baruch, G., Hickey, N., & Fonagy, P. (2011). A randomized controlled trial of multisystemic therapy and a statutory therapeutic intervention for young offenders. *Journal of the American Academy of Child & Adolescent Psychiatry, 50*(12), 1220–1235.

Caldwell, M., Skeem, J., Salekin, R., & Van Rybroek, G. (2006). Treatment response of adolescent offenders with psychopathy features a 2-year follow-up. *Criminal Justice and Behavior, 33*(5), 571–596.

Cauffman, E., Feldman, S., Watherman, J., & Steiner, H. (1998). Posttraumatic stress disorder among female juvenile offenders. *Journal of the American Academy of Child & Adolescent Psychiatry, 37*(11), 1209–1216.

Cauffman, E., Kimonis, E. R., Dmitrieva, J., & Monahan, K. C. (2009). A multimethod assessment of juvenile psychopathy: comparing the predictive utility of the PCL: YV, YPI, and NEO PRI. *Psychological Assessment, 21*(4), 528–542.

Cauffman, E., & Steinberg, L. (2000). (Im) maturity of judgment in adolescence: Why adolescents may be less culpable than adults. *Behavioral Sciences & the Law, 18*(6), 741–760.

Cauffman, E., Steinberg, L., & Piquero, A. R. (2005). Psychological, neuropsychological and physiological correlates of serious antisocial behavior in adolescence: The role of self-control. *Criminology, 43*(1), 133–176.

Celio, M., Karnik, N. S., & Steiner, H. (2006). Early maturation as a risk factor for aggression and delinquency in adolescent girls: A review. *International Journal of Clinical Practice, 60*(10), 1254–1262.

Chu, C. M., & Thomas, S. D. (2010). Adolescent sexual offenders: The relationship between typology and recidivism. *Sexual Abuse: A Journal of Research and Treatment, 22*(2), 218–233.

Cicchetti, D., & Rogosch, F. A. (1996). Equifinality and multifinality in developmental psychopathology. *Development and Psychopathology, 8*(4), 597–600.

Corrado, R. R., Vincent, G. M., Hart, S. D., & Cohen, I. M. (2004). Predictive validity of the Psychopathy Checklist: Youth Version for general and violent recidivism. *Behavioral Sciences & the Law, 22*(1), 5–22.

Costa, P. T., & McCrae, R. R. (1988). Personality in adulthood: A six-year longitudinal study of self-reports and spouse ratings on the NEO Personality Inventory. *Journal of Personality and Social Psychology, 54*(5), 853–863.

De Haan, L. G., & MacDermid, S. M. (1999). Identity development as a mediating factor between urban poverty and behavioral outcomes for junior high school students. *Journal of Family and Economic Issues, 20*(2), 123–148.

Dishion, T. J., McCord, J., & Poulin, F. (1999). When interventions harm: Peer groups and problem behavior. *American Psychologist, 54*(9), 755–764.

Fagan, J., & Deschenes, E. P. (1990). Determinants of judicial waiver decisions for violent juvenile offenders. *Journal of Criminal Law & Criminology, 81*(2), 314–347.

Feldman, S. S., & Weinberger, D. A. (1994). Self-restraint as a mediator of family influences on boys' delinquent behavior: A longitudinal study. *Child Development, 65*(1), 195–211.

Fine, A., Steinberg, L., Frick, P. J., & Cauffman, E. (2016). Self-control assessments and implications for predicting adolescent offending. *Journal of Youth and Adolescence, 45*(4), 701–712.

Fo, W. S., & O'Donnell, C. R. (1975). The buddy system: Effect of community intervention on delinquent offenses. *Behavior Therapy, 6*(4), 522–524.

Forth, A. E., Kosson, D. S., Hare, R. D., Sevecke, K., & Krischer, M. K. (2014). *Hare Psychopathy Checklist, Youth Version: PCL: YV.* Helsinki: Hogrefe.

Frick, P. J., Kimonis, E. R., Dandreaux, D. M., & Farell, J. M. (2003). The 4 year stability of psychopathic traits in non-referred youth. *Behavioral Sciences & the Law, 21*(6), 713–736.

Gillis, A. J., & Bath, E. (2016). Demographics. *Child and Adolescent Psychiatric Clinics of North America, 25*(1), 1–17.

Goodwill, A. M., Alison, L. J., & Beech, A. R. (2009). What works in offender profiling? A comparison of typological, thematic, and multivariate models. *Behavioral Sciences & the Law, 27*(4), 507–529.

Grisso, T., Steinberg, L., Woolard, J., Cauffman, E., Scott, E., Graham, S., ... Schwartz, R. (2003). Juveniles' competence to stand trial: A comparison of adolescents' and adults' capacities as trial defendants. *Law and Human Behavior, 27*(4), 333–363.

Groth, A. N., Burgess, W., & Holmstrom, L. L. (1977). Rape: Power, anger, and sexuality. *The American Journal of Psychiatry, 134*(11), 1239–1243. doi:10.1176/ajp.134.11.1239

Hare, R. D., & Vertommen, H. (1991). *The Hare Psychopathy Checklist–revised.* North Tonawanda, NY: Multi-Health Systems.

Harris, G. T., Rice, M. E., & Cormier, C. A. (1991). Psychopathy and violent recidivism. *Law and Human Behavior, 15*(6), 625–637.

Hawes, D. J., Price, M. J., & Dadds, M. R. (2014). Callous-unemotional traits and the treatment of conduct problems in childhood and adolescence: A comprehensive review. *Clinical Child and Family Psychology Review, 17*(3), 248–267.

Hazelwood, R. R. (1987). Analyzing the rape and profiling the offender. In R. R. Hazelwood & A. W. Burgess (Eds.), *Practical aspects of rape investigation: A multidisciplinary approach* (pp. 169–199). Boca Raton, FL: CRC Press.

Hazelwood, R. R., Ressler, R. K., Depue, R. L., & Douglas, J. C. (1995). Criminal investigative analysis: An overview. In R. R. Hazelwood & A. W. Burgess (Eds.), *Practical aspects of rape investigation: A multidisciplinary approach* (pp. 115–126). Boca Raton, FL: CRC Press.

Henggeler, S. W. (2012). Multisystemic therapy: Clinical foundations and research outcomes. *Psychosocial Intervention, 21*(2), 181–193.

Henggeler, S. W., Melton, G. B., & Smith, L. A. (1992). Family preservation using multisystemic therapy: An effective alternative to incarcerating serious juvenile offenders. *Journal of Consulting and Clinical Psychology, 60*(6), 953–961.

Henggeler, S. W., & Sheidow, A. J. (2012). Empirically supported family-based treatments for conduct disorder and delinquency in adolescents. *Journal of Marital and Family Therapy, 38*(1), 30–58.

Huckaby, W. J., Kohler, M., Garner, E. H., & Steiner, H. (1998). A comparison between the Weinberger Adjustment Inventory and the Minnesota Multiphasic Personality Inventory with incarcerated adolescent males. *Child Psychiatry and Human Development, 28*(4), 273–285.

Johnson, J. L., & Johnson, C. F. (2001). Poverty and the death penalty. *Journal of Economic Issues, 35*(2), 517–523.

Karnik, N. S., McMullin, M. A., & Steiner, H. (2006). Disruptive behaviors: Conduct and oppositional disorders in adolescents. *Adolescent Medicine Clinics, 17*(1), 97–114.

Karnik, N. S., Soller, M., Redlich, A., Silverman, M., Kraemer, H. C., Haapanen, R., & Steiner, H. (2009). Prevalence of and gender differences in psychiatric disorders among juvenile delinquents incarcerated for nine months. *Psychiatric Services, 60*(6), 838–841.

Karnik, N. S., Soller, M. V., Redlich, A., Silverman, M. A., Kraemer, H. C., Haapanen, R., & Steiner, H. (2010). Prevalence differences of psychiatric disorders among youth after nine months or more of incarceration by race/ethnicity and age. *Journal of Health Care for the Poor and Underserved, 21*(1), 237–250.

Karnik, N. S., & Steiner, H. (2007). Evidence for interventions for young offenders. *Child and Adolescent Mental Health, 12*(4), 154–159.

Kaszynski, K., Kallis, D. L., Karnik, N., Soller, M., Hunter, S., Haapanen, R., ... Steiner, H. (2014). Incarcerated youth with personality disorders: Prevalence, comorbidity and convergent validity. *Personality and Mental Health, 8*(1), 42–51.

Kleck, G. (1981). Racial discrimination in criminal sentencing: A critical evaluation of the evidence with additional evidence on the death penalty. *American Sociological Review, 46*(6), 783–805.

Klietz, S. J., Borduin, C. M., & Schaeffer, C. M. (2010). Cost–benefit analysis of multisystemic therapy with serious and violent juvenile offenders. *Journal of Family Psychology, 24*(5), 657–666.

Kolko, D. J., & Pardini, D. A. (2010). ODD dimensions, ADHD, and callous–unemotional traits as predictors of treatment response in children with disruptive behavior disorders. *Journal of Abnormal Psychology, 119*(4), 713–725.

Kosson, D. S., Cyterski, T. D., Steuerwald, B. L., Neumann, C. S., & Walker-Matthews, S. (2002). The reliability and validity of the Psychopathy Checklist: Youth Version (PCL: YV) in non-incarcerated adolescent males. *Psychological Assessment, 14*(1), 97–109.

Lembke, A. (2013). When it comes to addiction, the DSM-5 gets it right, but . . . New York: Pacific Standard. https://psmag.com/when-it-comes-to-addiction-the-dsm-5-gets-it-right-but-e3edc153182f#.22qv30jfe

Levinson, J. D., Smith, R. J., & Young, D. M. (2014). Devaluing death: An empirical study of implicit racial bias on jury-eligible citizens in six death penalty states. *New York University Law Review, 89*, 513. (pages 1–65)

Levintova, H. (2015). Girls are the fastest-growing group in the juvenile justice system. *Mother Jones.* http://www.motherjones.com/politics/2015/09/girls-make-ever-growing-proportion-kids-juvenile-justice-system

Lipsey, M. W. (2006). The effects of community-based group treatment for delinquency. In K. A. Dodge; T. J. Dishion, & J. E. Lansford (Eds.), *Deviant peer influences in programs for youth: Problems and solutions* (pp. 162–184). New York: Guilford Press.

Lussier, P., McCuish, E., & Corrado, R. R. (2015). The adolescence–adulthood transition and desistance from crime: Examining the underlying structure of desistance. *Journal of Developmental and Life-Course Criminology, 1*(2), 87–117.

Lynam, D. R., Caspi, A., Moffitt, T. E., Loeber, R., & Stouthamer-Loeber, M. (2007). Longitudinal evidence that psychopathy scores in early adolescence predict adult psychopathy. *Journal of Abnormal Psychology, 116*(1), 155–165.

McCollister, K. E., French, M. T., & Fang, H. (2010). The cost of crime to society: New crime-specific estimates for policy and program evaluation. *Drug and Alcohol Dependence, 108*(1), 98–109.

Merriam-Webster. (2006). *Merriam-Webster's dictionary of law.* Springfield, MA: Author.

Miller, A. K., Rufino, K. A., Boccaccini, M. T., Jackson, R. L., & Murrie, D. C. (2011). On individual differences in person perception: Raters' personality traits relate to their Psychopathy Checklist-Revised scoring tendencies. *Assessment, 18*(2), 253–260.

Moffitt, T. E., Arseneault, L., Belsky, D., Dickson, N., Hancox, R. J., Harrington, H., . . . Ross, S. (2011). A gradient of childhood self-control predicts health, wealth, and public safety. *Proceedings of the National Academy of Sciences, 108*(7), 2693–2698.

Mulder, E., Vermunt, J., Brand, E., Bullens, R., & Marle, H. (2012). Recidivism in subgroups of serious juvenile offenders: Different profiles, different risks? *Criminal Behaviour and Mental Health, 22*(2), 122–135.

Mulvey, E. P. (2011). *Highlights from pathways to desistance: A longitudinal study of serious adolescent offenders.* Washington, DC: Office of Juvenile Justice and Delinquency Prevention, US Department of Justice.

Murrie, D. C., Boccaccini, M. T., Guarnera, L. A., & Rufino, K. A. (2013). Are forensic experts biased by the side that retained them? *Psychological Science, 24*(10), 1889–1897.

Murrie, D. C., Boccaccini, M. T., Turner, D. B., Meeks, M., Woods, C., & Tussey, C. (2009). Rater (dis)agreement on risk assessment measures in sexually violent predator proceedings: Evidence of adversarial allegiance in forensic evaluation? *Psychology, Public Policy, and Law, 15*(1), 19. (pages 1889–1897)

Newcomb, M. D., & Bentler, P. M. (1989). Substance use and abuse among children and teenagers. *American Psychologist, 44*(2), 242–248.

Odgers, C. L., Reppucci, N. D., & Moretti, M. M. (2005). Nipping psychopathy in the bud: An examination of the convergent, predictive, and theoretical utility of the PCL-YV among adolescent girls. *Behavioral Sciences & the Law, 23*(6), 743–763.

Office of Juvenile Justice and Delinquency Prevention. (2015). Statistica briefing book. https://www.ojjdp.gov/ojstatbb/

Piquero, A. R. (2008). Disproportionate minority contact. *The Future of Children, 18*(2), 59–79.

Plattner, B., Giger, J., Bachmann, F., Brühwiler, K., Steiner, H., Steinhausen, H.-C., . . . Aebi, M. (2012). Psychopathology and offense types in detained male juveniles. *Psychiatry Research, 198*(2), 285–290.

Plattner, B., Kraemer, H. C., Williams, R. P., Bauer, S. M., Kindler, J., Feucht, M., . . . Steiner, H. (2007). Suicidality, psychopathology, and gender in incarcerated adolescents in Austria. *Journal of Clinical Psychiatry, 68*(10), 1593–1600.

Plattner, B., Steiner, H., The, S. S., Kraemer, H. C., Bauer, S. M., Kindler, J., . . . Feucht, M. (2009). Sex-specific predictors of criminal recidivism in a representative sample of incarcerated youth. *Comprehensive Psychiatry, 50*(5), 400–407.

Prentky, R., & Righthand, S. (2003). *Juvenile sex offender assessment protocol-II (J-SOAP-II) manual.* Washington, DC: US Department of Justice, Office of Justice Programs, Office of Juvenile Justice and Delinquency Prevention.

Pullman, L., & Seto, M. C. (2012). Assessment and treatment of adolescent sexual offenders: Implications of recent research on generalist versus specialist explanations. *Child Abuse & Neglect, 36*(3), 203–209.

Rhiner, B., Graf, T., Dammann, G., & Fuerstenau, U. (2011). [Multisystemic Therapy (MST) for adolescents with severe conduct disorders in German-speaking Switzerland-implementation and first results]. *Zeitschrift für Kinder-und Jugendpsychiatrie und Psychotherapie, 39*(1), 33–39.

Rice, M. E., & Harris, G. T. (2013). Psychopathy and violent recidivism. In K. A. Kiehl & W. Sinnott-Armstrong (Eds.), *Handbook on psychopathy and law* (pp. 231–249). Oxford: Oxford University Press.

Santisteban, D. A., Coatsworth, J. D., Perez-Vidal, A., Kurtines, W. M., Schwartz, S. J., LaPerriere, A., & Szapocznik, J. (2003). Efficacy of brief strategic family therapy in modifying Hispanic adolescent behavior problems and substance use. *Journal of Family Psychology, 17*(1), 121–133.

Schmidt, F., Campbell, M. A., & Houlding, C. (2011). Comparative analyses of the YLS/CMI, SAVRY, and PCL: YV in adolescent offenders: A 10-year follow-up into adulthood. *Youth Violence and Juvenile Justice, 9*(1), 23–42.

Schmidt, F., McKinnon, L., Chattha, H. K., & Brownlee, K. (2006). Concurrent and predictive validity of the Psychopathy Checklist: Youth Version across gender and ethnicity. *Psychological Assessment, 18*(4), 393–401.

Schoenwald, S. K., Ward, D. M., Henggeler, S. W., Pickrel, S. G., & Patel, H. (1996). Multisystemic therapy treatment of substance abusing or dependent adolescent offenders: Costs of reducing incarceration, inpatient, and residential placement. *Journal of Child and Family Studies, 5*(4), 431–444.

Scott, E. S., & Steinberg, L. D. (2009). *Rethinking juvenile justice.* Cambridge, MA: Harvard University Press.

Sheidow, A. J., Bradford, W. D., Henggeler, S. W., Rowland, M. D., Halliday-Boykins, C., Schoenwald, S. K., & Ward, D. M. (2004). Treatment costs for youths receiving multisystemic therapy or hospitalization after a psychiatric crisis. *Psychiatric Services, 55*(5), 548–554.

Shelton, D., Kesten, K., Zhang, W., & Trestman, R. (2011). Impact of a dialectic behavior therapy—Corrections Modified (DBT-CM) upon behaviorally challenged incarcerated male adolescents. *Journal of Child and Adolescent Psychiatric Nursing, 24*(2), 105–113.

Shepherd, S. M., & Strand, S. (2016). The utility of the Psychopathy Checklist: Youth Version (PCL: YV) and the Youth Psychopathic Trait Inventory (YPI)—Is it meaningful to measure psychopathy in young offenders? *Psychological assessment, 28*(4), 405–415.

Sherman, F., & Balck, A. (2015). Gender injustice: System-level juvenile justice reforms for girls. http://nationalcrittenton.org/wp-content/uploads/2015/09/GenderInjustice_exec_summary.pdf

Shrier, L. A., Harris, S. K., Kurland, M., & Knight, J. R. (2003). Substance use problems and associated psychiatric symptoms among adolescents in primary care. *Pediatrics, 111*(6), e699–e705.

Snook, B., Cullen, R. M., Bennell, C., Taylor, P. J., & Gendreau, P. (2008). The criminal profiling illusion: What's behind the smoke and mirrors? *Criminal Justice and Behavior, 35*(10), 1257–1276.

Stedman, T. L. (2006). *Stedman's medical dictionary.* Baltimore: Lippincott Williams & Wilkins.

Steinberg, L., Albert, D., Cauffman, E., Banich, M., Graham, S., & Woolard, J. (2008). Age differences in sensation seeking and impulsivity as indexed by behavior and self-report: Evidence for a dual systems model. *Developmental Psychology, 44*(6), 1764–1778.

Steinberg, L., & Scott, E. S. (2003). Less guilty by reason of adolescence: Developmental immaturity, diminished responsibility, and the juvenile death penalty. *American psychologist, 58*(12), 1009–1018.

Steiner, H. (1997). Practice parameters for the assessment and treatment of children and adolescents with conduct disorder. *Journal of the American Academy of Child & Adolescent Psychiatry, 36*(10), 122S–139S.

Steiner, H., & Cauffman, E. (1998). Juvenile justice, delinquency, and psychiatry. *Child and Adolescent Psychiatric Clinics of North America, 7*(3), 653–672.

Steiner, H., Cauffman, E., & Duxbury, E. (1999). Personality traits in juvenile delinquents: Relation to criminal behavior and recidivism. *Journal of the American Academy of Child & Adolescent Psychiatry, 38*(3), 256–262. doi:10.1097/00004583-199903000-00011

Steiner, H., & Hall, R. E. (2015). *Treating adolescents.* Hoboken, NJ: John Wiley.

Steiner, H., Humphreys, K., & Redlich, A. (2001). *The assessment of the mental health system of the California Youth Authority: Report to Governor Gray Davis.* Stanford, CA: Stanford University.

Steiner, H., Silverman, M., Karnik, N. S., Huemer, J., Plattner, B., Clark, C. E., . . . Haapanen, R. (2011). Psychopathology, trauma and delinquency: Subtypes of aggression and their relevance for understanding young offenders. *Child and Adolescent Psychiatry and Mental Health, 5*(1), 21. (11 total pages)

Swogger, M. T., Walsh, Z., Christie, M., Priddy, B. M., & Conner, K. R. (2015). Impulsive versus premeditated aggression in the prediction of violent criminal recidivism. *Aggressive Behavior, 41*(4), 346–352.

Szapocznik, J., & Prado, G. (2007). Negative effects on family functioning from psychosocial treatments: A recommendation for expanded safety monitoring. *Journal of Family Psychology, 21*(3), 468–478.

Tapia, M. (2010). Untangling race and class effects on juvenile arrests. *Journal of Criminal Justice, 38*(3), 255–265.

Teplin, L. A., Abram, K. M., McClelland, G. M., Dulcan, M. K., & Mericle, A. A. (2002). Psychiatric disorders in youth in juvenile detention. *Archives of General Psychiatry, 59*(12), 1133–1143.

Teplin, L. A., Abram, K. M., Washburn, J. J., Welty, L. J., Hershfield, J. A., & Dulcan, M. K. (2013). The Northwestern Juvenile Project: Overview. *Juvenile Justice Bulletin, 13.* (or pages 1–16)

Terracciano, A., McCrae, R. R., & Costa, P. T. (2010). Intra-individual change in personality stability and age. *Journal of Research in Personality, 44*(1), 31–37.

van der Stouwe, T., Asscher, J. J., Stams, G. J. J., Deković, M., & van der Laan, P. H. (2014). The effectiveness of Multisystemic Therapy (MST): A meta-analysis. *Clinical Psychology Review, 34*(6), 468–481.

Vazsonyi, A. T., & Chen, P. (2010). Entry risk into the juvenile justice system: African American, American Indian, Asian American, European American, and Hispanic children and adolescents. *Journal of Child Psychology and Psychiatry, 51*(6), 668–678.

Wagner, D. V., Borduin, C. M., Sawyer, A. M., & Dopp, A. R. (2014). Long-term prevention of criminality in siblings of serious and violent juvenile offenders: A 25-year follow-up to a randomized clinical trial of multisystemic therapy. *Journal of Consulting and Clinical Psychology, 82*(3), 492–499.

Weinberger, D., Feldman, S., Ford, M., & Chastain, R. (1987). Construct validation of the Weinberger Adjustment Inventory. Unpublished manuscript, Stanford University.

Weinberger, D. A., & Schwartz, G. E. (1990). Distress and restraint as superordinate dimensions of self-reported adjustment: A typological perspective. *Journal of Personality, 58*(2), 381–417.

Weiss, B., Caron, A., Ball, S., Tapp, J., Johnson, M., & Weisz, J. R. (2005). Iatrogenic effects of group treatment for antisocial youths. *Journal of Consulting and Clinical Psychology, 73*(6), 1036–1044.

Wilson, C. R., Sherritt, L., Gates, E., & Knight, J. R. (2004). Are clinical impressions of adolescent substance use accurate? *Pediatrics, 114*(5), e536–e540.

Suggested Reading and Resources

Aichorn, A. (1935). *Wayward youth.* New York: Viking Press.

Benedek, E. P., Ash, P., & Scott, C. L. (Eds.). (2009). *Principles and practice of child and adolescent forensic mental health.* Washington, DC: American Psychiatric Publishing.

Grisso, T. (1998). *Forensic evaluation of juveniles.* Sarasota, FL: Professional Resource Press.

Hubner, J., & Wolfson, J. (2003). *Somebody else's children: The courts, the kids, and the struggle to save America's troubled families.* New York: Authors Choice Press.

Humes, E. (2015). *No matter how loud I shout: A year in the life of juvenile court.* New York: Simon & Schuster.

Scott, E. S., & Steinberg, L. D. (2009). *Rethinking juvenile justice.* Cambridge, MA: Harvard University Press.

7

Summary and Epilogue

In this, our final chapter we briefly summarize what we have learned in each of the previous chapters and then give a glimpse into the future of this important field, that is, the study of disruptive behavior disorders (DBDs), their diagnosis, and their treatment. The following is a simple account that will demonstrate the considerable growth in this specific field of developmental psychopathology. When one of the authors (HS) wrote the American Academy of Child & Adolescent Psychology practice parameter for conduct disorders (CDs) in 1997, he reviewed over 1,000 books, chapters, and peer-reviewed papers. While the literature was voluminous, the quantity was driven mostly by information published in criminology, while studies from a medical-psychiatric point of view were lacking. The literature at that time portrayed a skewed picture: samples used were predominantly incarcerated, male, ethnic minorities of poor economic background. Not surprisingly, violence and drug-related crimes were overrepresented. In reviewing the literature one came away with the impression that DBDs were a problem of the poor, male, ethnic minorities in special facilities designed to contain, punish, and sometimes educate and rehabilitate. In light of these circumstances, a deliberate attempt was made for the practice parameter to focus on studies with greater ecological, medical, and external validity—studies that at that time were in the minority. The practice parameter called for a change in theoretical basis (developmental psychopathology and psychiatry) and broader-based, more representative studies in the general and in clinical populations.

In 2007 the same author (HS) wrote the oppositional defiant disorder (ODD) practice parameter. Identical key words were used for literature searches, and, like that of the searches performed 10 years prior, over 1,000 articles, books, and book chapters were reviewed. However, this time, 81% of the sources came from child, adolescent, and developmental psychiatry with only 19% of the sources having been published in the field of criminology. These medical and criminological data made it clear that juvenile justice settings had become the psychiatric and mental health clinics for poor youth in need of intensive services, hardly a laudable finding. The governors of California were made aware of this fact and, to their credit, began to implement some of the crucial changes the Stanford/NIJ/CYA project had suggested in 2001 and 2002. In addition, some of the changes called for in the CDs practice parameter from 10 years prior had taken place and were reported in the medical literature. There was finally enough information to begin to distribute results and findings across three relevant domains in developmental psychiatry: biological, psychological, and social. At the same time, there was persistent agreement among the major authors in the field that any single factor causal model would not serve us well in the study, diagnosis, and treatment of DBDs. Multifactorial models needed to be developed and tested in further studies.

During the writing of this book, it has once again become clear that although far from being in an ideal situation, considerable progress has occurred. Utilizing the same search terms as in previous years for our preparatory searches on Medline, PsychINFO, and other scholarly search engines yielded a vast literature base—a literature base that has begun to report studies utilizing the most cutting-edge medical instrumentation, such as imaging, genetic studies, and studies linking phenotypes (i.e. what we see as parents, clinicians, and researchers) and underlying processes contributing to the risk for emergence, persistence, and desistence of DBDs. We have come a long way from the Chicago reformers and August Aichhorn. Here we summarize and highlight some of the specifics in each subdomain of study of DBDs as contained in all of the previous chapters of this book. This chapter may serve as a guidepost and source of inspiration and encouragement for the next generations of clinicians, researchers, parents, and their children afflicted by DBDs.

In chapter 1, "Introduction to Disruptive Behavior Disorders," we recapitulated the history of bringing medicine, development, psychology, and forensics together in an ongoing effort to assist and heal those who suffer from a range of predominantly externalizing disorders. We went over the historical events that provided the major impetus to view problems with laws, antisocial acts, and aggression from the point of view of medicine. The Chicago reformers deserve most of the credit for starting this line of thinking and changing the way the law deals with youths who have committed crimes. August Aichhorn brought to these problems the idea that development and psychology play an important role in the pathogenesis of crime and the idea that psychoeducation, therapy, and treatment could alter the course of these youths' life trajectories. We began to sketch the demands placed on these diagnoses in order for them to be of use clinically. This required us to examine the validity of the diagnostic constructs used to characterize these youths, in addition to their relationship to normal development and psychopathology. Our work also compelled us to elucidate the relationship DBD diagnoses have to putative causal mechanisms. In doing so, we hoped to address anticipated scrutiny by lawmakers, juvenile justice workers, and interested lay persons, thereby laying the groundwork for a detailed discussion of DBD diagnoses in chapter 2.

In chapter 2, "Taxonomy, Classification, and Diagnosis of Disruptive Behavior Disorders," we presented a comprehensive overview and comparison of the diagnostic labels used for grouping DBDs. A great deal of discussion was dedicated to elucidating the professional activities and processes leading up to the current DBD diagnoses. We also examined the theoretical basis of these labels, their criteria, and the data supporting the taxonomies generated. Such scrutiny has been driven for many years by the multiple critical voices that have arisen within the fields of psychiatry and psychology, related researchers, and the lay public. It is of critical importance that our profession be ready to discuss clinical and research problems with these diagnostic labels whenever we bring the worlds of medicine and criminal justice together. We must be fully aware of both the utility and the limitations of the descriptive diagnostic systems currently prevalent in psychiatric medicine, so as to not end up overselling or underselling what medicine has to offer in this important dialogue. The world the physician and mental health worker enters in diagnosing, treating, and studying delinquency and crime from a medical perspective is not necessarily welcoming, supportive, and receptive. We have to be prepared to encounter resistance and justified criticism on multiple fronts.

In this taxonomy and diagnosis chapter, we hope to have conveyed the complexity and uncertainty that arises when we attempt to describe the assumed internal disturbance associated with aggressive and antisocial behavior. Our field is placed in a rather difficult position when describing and seeking to diagnose mental disorders associated with such externalizing behaviors from a medical-psychiatric point of view. This is because the DBD criteria must require another person to be involved, not just one's own internal subjective experience (e.g., when is taking a pen from someone stealing and when is it justified reappropriation?). This is quite different from the criteria for many internalizing disorders (e.g., depression, anxiety), which are primarily based on an individual's self-reported experience, from the patient's point of view. More simply put, externalizing disorders such as DBDs in almost all their constituent criteria directly or indirectly need another person or persons to be present in some form to make the criterion work. Such reliance on interpersonal interactions in formulating DBD diagnoses immediately begs the question of contextual variables that can drive disease processes. Our current taxonomy and array of diagnoses continue to struggle to address the influence of context (e.g., genetic, temperament, family, community) on the development and diagnosis itself of DBDs in a decisive way. Such difficulties persist despite the considerable progress our field has made in developing a professional consensus regarding the best descriptors and medical terms for externalizing disorders. We will need continued creativity and thought around resolving the issue of, for instance, when is stealing, lying, attacking others, resisting laws and refusing to follow them justified and not a sign of psychiatric disorder, which is predominantly internally driven? When do problems like DBDs exculpate the patient, or when can DBDs be used as good indicators for specific interventions that will lead to rehabilitation and healing? Such questions remain largely unanswered. We need to resolve these issues to avoid stigmatization and wrongful exculpation of the individuals involved. The world of law needs us to be certain when we call an antisocial act an illness versus a violation of laws governing our conduct.

There are multiple problems with various forms of validity of DBD diagnoses. DBDs in their current iteration remain imprecise and heterogenous, indicating issues with discriminant validity and, possibly, construct validity. Their diagnostic criteria's strength of cohesion is unknown. Furthermore, the prospective validity of DBDs is poor and may not have been adequately tested. There is some support for concurrent validity, which emerges from studies of multiple observers using the criteria independently and blindly. In our experience, working with young professionals in training as raters for the Stanford/NIJ/CYA projects, indicators of agreement were low to moderate and not easily achieved or maintained.

Such uncertainties have fueled a long debate in the relevant literature about how to best capture DBDs, among other mental problems—categorical (diagnosis) versus dimensional (traits and states). Both have advantages and disadvantages: diagnoses are types that summarize a great deal of information and facilitate rapid communication between professionals. The main drawback of diagnoses is that they can become overgeneralized stereotypes leading to rubberstamping and stigma. Also, it is rarely the case that all patients with a given diagnosis are the same, especially when diagnoses are relative newcomers or are based on a problematic theory. In DBDs there are usually a whole host of factors operative in the background that are not captured but have important influences—for example, nutritional status, pediatric health and chronic illnesses, or toxic influences substances such as lead.

Dimensional approaches do not assume discontinuity between diagnosis and normalcy. They seek to capture patient characteristics along a continuum. This offers the advantage to the clinician that certain traits can be targeted long before a special diagnosis is established, ideally leading to early intervention and even prevention. Dimensions can deliver a finer-grained picture of moderators and mediators of disease, in addition to comorbidity subtypes. This approach is very much in line with developmental thinking, which is most appropriate for changing organisms, such as youths.

The problem with the dimensional approach, which is more at home in psychology than medicine, is that information from multiple dimensions is difficult to convey and base rapid decisions on, something that doctors need to do expediently on a daily basis. In the end, the most prudent approach, given the current state of knowledge and our current taxonomy of antisocial behavior and aggression, is to combine dimensional and typological assessment. To establish a diagnosis provides a basis for necessary next steps. These next steps are then based on subtypes of diagnoses (such as early onset vs. late onset CD) and subdividing dimensions (such as callous–unemotional traits). This is entirely in line with the thinking in the rest of medicine. We increasingly realize that not all patients with a certain disease (e.g., breast cancer) are created equal: we need to go beyond diagnosis to subtypes and dimensions to deliver precision health. In the case of DBDs, we are very much in the same position, with an important message to pass on to our next generation of students, researchers, and practitioners.

The International Classification of Diseases (ICD) and the *Diagnostic and Statistical Manual of Mental Disorders* (DSM) are probably best thought of as tools of communication between practitioners and insurance companies. The original intent to provide a tool for research has failed, at least as far as DBDs are concerned. As we started to outline earlier, we recommend that the DSM or ICD labels be used as a start to the clinical process but that following reaching a descriptive diagnosis we go further, beneath the surface, and look for causal loops and processes that keep these disorders going. These variables can arise at any level of the biopsychosocial continuum. These factors seem to unfold over years starting at birth. When they reach a critical threshold, risk becomes disorder. This thinking derives from developmental psychopathology, which sees DBDs, especially CD, as a paradigmatic condition. While this model can be problematic due to its inherent complexity, it also holds a promise to be helpful in the long run by avoiding premature reductionism and orthodoxy.

We end chapter 2 by providing a possible new grouping of DBDs along a normalcy/disorder spectrum. We also suggest this new grouping be based on the important distinction between antisocial and/or aggressive events of an emotionally charged and emotionally cold nature. Such distinctions (e.g., hot vs. cold, impulsive vs. premeditated) were originally derived from a legal and justice perspective but have become increasingly supported by findings in neuroscience (discussed in chapter 4 on etiology). We have come to a point where we could provide a taxonomy for DBDs that has immediate clinical implications and is in line with legal codices that are increasingly supported by neuroscientific findings.

In chapter 3, "Epidemiology of Disruptive Behavior Disorders," we discuss the available best empirical support for the occurrence and prevalence of DBDs in different samples in either clinics, the general population, or justice settings. Simply put, the available epidemiological evidence is very uneven. Some of the unevenness is created by the changes in the DBD criteria between DSM updates. Progress has been made in making the ICD and the DSM systems more consonant, but the grouping s of DBDs in the two systems remains quite different. Such differences carry both advantages and disadvantages, which ultimately will have to be settled by empirical studies. At the present time there is no ideal and complete study of the epidemiology of DBDs, or even for a single one of the included diagnostic categories. As we discussed, such ideal studies are tripartite studies, going from basic screens to specific instruments followed by in-depth clinical assessments of systematically selected high and low scorers on the basic screens. The lack of epidemiological data is particularly apparent in the newly added diagnoses (e.g. pyromania, kleptomania, etc.). There are some new and interesting longitudinal studies of DBDs, which carry extra weight because of their prospective design with high levels of retention of participants from baseline to follow-up points.

In sum, studies confirm the relatively high prevalence of some DBDs in different populations, not just incarcerative settings. Overall, there is progress in the epidemiology of DBDs that seems to map onto the clinical impression that these disorders are very common and complicated; however, we remain far from the multiple converging lines of epidemiologic evidence needed to glimpse the causal processes of DBDs. In our view, the repeated switching of criteria for DBDs, driven by committee rather than data, continues to interfere with the collection of needed long-term and consistent data. This is yet another reason why the introduction of the research domain criteria by the National Institute for Mental Health might be an excellent step in the right direction, as one would hope that this taxonomy would be studied and made more valid by scientific study, not secret committee work.

The main remaining issue in DBDs' epidemiology is arriving at some precise understanding of the effect of having changed the criteria for DBDs repeatedly over the past few decades. The net change from the vantage point of the current iteration of the diagnoses seems to be an increasingly longer list of criteria to which severity and frequency specifiers have been added. This could of course lead to beneficial outcomes, such as an increase in precision and various forms of validity, but such benefits are not guaranteed and remain to be seen in comparative studies. The addition of new dimensional subtypes (callous–unemotional in CD, for instance) is encouraging and in line with the thinking in developmental psychiatry. It should help clinicians arrive at a better starting position as they prepare to intervene.

Information is needed across almost all the constituent diagnoses in the DBD grouping. It would also be important to report on the impact of the repeated changes of the DBD grouping itself and comparisons that help us decide which grouping—ICD versus DSM—might be most logical and impactful. ICD remains different from DSM in this regard. The ICD grouping implicitly and explicitly contains some ways of creating DBD subtypes that have some utility in clinical practice and possibly research.

Another still unsettled issue is the exact relationship of the DBD diagnoses to each other. The question, as to whether ODD and CD, for instance, are separate disorders altogether or are on a continuum, with ODD being an intrafamilial precursor to CD, is unanswered. The DSM keeps changing in its position on this issue without showing the empirical support for such changes. The ICD's position to have ODD be a subtype—a forerunner of CD—makes more sense from the standpoint of developmental psychopathology.

Yet another open question concerns the proper representation of how DBDs are related to other categories of psychopathology. There are many studies reporting a frequent co-occurrence of DBDs with neuropsychiatric syndromes, such as autism, intellectual disability, attention deficit hyperactivity disorder (ADHD) and learning problems, internalizing disorders such as anxiety and mood disorders, and substance and alcohol use in mild, moderate, and severe forms. All these have important clinical implications, which have only become more pressing, as psychiatric treatment has evolved and become increasingly effective and specific. But the taxonomies still struggle with how to best understand this frequent co-occurrence: Are we dealing with disorders that are truly separate and co-incidental? Or are we better off thinking about some of these problems as being part of DBDs? Again, the ICD and DSM diverge on how to approach this problem. Whether one or the other way is preferable is an issue to be settled soon for us to achieve deeper understanding of DBDs and better treatment outcomes. The DSM favors a separate disease–comorbidity model. The ICD tends to see these conditions as common accompaniments of DBDs, which can be used to subtypify. The ICD approach is more in line with findings from the neuroscience literature, which increasingly show the enormous connectivity of brain regions seemingly dedicated to different and separate functions. Such a theoretical posture fits better with a developmental psychiatry perspective that sees diagnoses as strongly influenced by age, maturation, and development. A "clean diagnosis" from such a point of view is a "developmental achievement." The presence of multiple disorders relates to immaturity and lack of differentiation more than the presence of massive psychopathology and comorbidity. The fact that up to 60% of DBDs also overlap with other externalizing disorders, such as substance use, might be a signal that underlying causal processes are shared and/or that diagnostic criteria should be amended to reflect this preponderant overlap. The same argument can also be made for the 40 or so percent overlap with internalizing disorders. This is another set of issues to settle more decisively if we are to achieve significant progress in DBDs.

In chapter 4, "Etiology of Disruptive Behavior Disorders," we find that our understanding of the etiology of DBDs is neither complete nor definitive. Such circumstances require that we continue to pay attention to factors from all three of the core domains relevant in developmental psychiatry: biological, psychological, and social. In order to facilitate understanding of such an array, we offer three ways of thinking about how to align and weigh information from these levels of abstraction. The levels range from subcellular factors all the way to family, community, and cultural environments. Each of these factors is capable of generating causal loops that lead to dysfunctions and DBDs. The Sroufe/Rutter tree of the developmental view of DBD diagnoses is an excellent aide in conceptualizing how genetic risk turns into a problem, which can be bypassed, be overcome, or lead to arrest or retreat from developmental progress. The risk/resilience factors scale model then helps us order this wide array of factors along a maturational continuum that assigns a different weight to a factor based on existing risk and age.

With this model in mind, we can examine the literature with greater clarity, offering many new leads in the three domains we consider crucial in the field of DBDs: biological, psychological, and social. The literature of relevant biological factors is growing, extending from the original neurotransmitter studies to genetic and epigenetic studies documenting vulnerabilities and risks. Many of the biological studies attempt to link peripheral measures of arousal in multiple channels (observable phenotypes) to activity in special central nervous system regions (endotypes that require special instrumentation to study and identify). Deficits in noradrenergic, serotonergic, and GABA-ergic neurotransmitters have been studies in DBDs in the 1980s up until 2016. To these data we have now added information regarding special genetic profiles that results in greater vulnerability in the context of abuse and stress. There are new and tantalizing links between the oxytocin system and problems with attachment and relationships so commonly found in DBDs. These same problems also seem to correlate with callous–unemotional traits. Furthermore, the literature on linking basic biological and psychological factors keeps expanding. There are several new studies linking behavioral observations to imaging of deficient brain systems. Psychological factors are also getting close to having implications for clinical practice, providing new tools for systematic screening and the development of specifically targeted treatments. Problems in learning and intelligence are repeatedly reported to contribute to the emergence of DBDs. There is an increase of positive findings regarding the different psychological accompaniments of emotionally "cold" and "hot" aggression, which influence the behavior of youth under stress. Fear extinction and conditioning are implicated in the genesis of antisocial and aggressive behavior, and these deficits seem to have special links to brain regions studied by imaging. The domain of social factors relevant to DBDs consistently supports a range of social influences of deviant development leading to DBDs. Families, parenting, media, neighborhoods, and physical environment are included among the factors that influence prosocial or antisocial development. Finally, using the label of psychopathy as a magnifying lens, we can see that all the factors mentioned continue to be of relevance in the pathogenesis of this most pernicious outcome in DBDs.

A clear-cut understanding of the etiology of DBDs is likely to remain out of our grasp for some years to come. For the time being, we can best characterize the pathogenesis of DBDs as a mosaic with many pieces still missing. Despite the remaining gaps in our knowledge, much progress has been made over the past 20 years. For instance, several meta-analyses have yielded broad -based support for some key concepts. Our current understanding of the causes of DBDs indicates that it is best to retain theories and disease models that combine biological/psychological and social factors, as we have outlined in this summary and in the chapter itself. We are increasingly able to detect and define processes that are involved in causal loops, ultimately to be targeted with specific interventions. Such an increase in our capacity to match treatment to pathogenic process will ultimately lead to more positive treatment outcomes.

In our opinion though, it will be developmental psychopathology approaches, rather than descriptive psychiatry, that will yield the most successful research and clinical practice in years to come. Our opinion is based on developmental psychiatry's emphasis on the multivariate causality of mental disorders, reliance on contextual analyses of symptoms, and pathogenic processes. Unlike descriptive psychiatry, developmental psychopathology acknowledges the continuum from normal to deviant development. Such an approach demands that we seek to understand the processes and causal factors underlying behavioral manifestations. In other words, developmental psychopathology seeks to connect theoretical modes with empiricism and scientific study in ways that mere descriptive approaches are not well equipped to do. We hope to have conveyed this fact by the case material at the end of chapter 4. All of these cases fulfilled current DSM and ICD criteria for a particular DBD. But as the case material shows, their pathway into these disorders could not have been more diverse. A rational taxonomy of DBDs must be able to accommodate such diversity among pathways in order to be helpful.

"Comprehensive and Integrated Treatment of Disruptive Behavior Disorders," chapter 5, shows a very large increment in higher quality studies independent of the criminological literature, but it is still fair to say that there is very uneven progress across the three subdomains of interventions: biological, psychological, and social. The strongest support, as has been true for the past 10 years or maybe more, is for the psychological/behavioral approaches, especially as far as ODD and CD are concerned. There are very few comparative studies of different psychological interventions, which are needed in order for the clinician to determine the more effective and efficacious treatments for the disorders in this grouping. A rare recent meta-analysis by Epstein, Fonnesbeck, Potter, Rizzone, and McPheeters (2015) set out to show differential effects of participants in therapy. The results supported the involvement of parents, regardless of age of the patient. This result once again speaks to the inherent complexity of DBDs: rarely, if ever, can we rely on individually based interventions alone, be they medications or therapy. The psychosocial components need to be thought about in targeted and integrated ways.

Another comprehensive review by Epstein et al. (2015) for the Agency for Healthcare Research and Quality shows us important facts to consider in medication treatment. As we have pointed out in our etiology and diagnosis chapters, the type of antisocial behavior and aggression determines many of the positive treatment effects of, for instance, antipsychotics and stimulants, as well as other forms of interventions: individuals with a high level of callous–unemotional traits were repeatedly shown to be much more treatment resistant. In turn, such individuals are very likely to have predominantly proactive/instrumental/ planned (PIP) type of antisocial and aggressive acts. This refractory response to intervention also extended to the psychosocial dimensions of treatment, as children with high levels of callous–unemotional traits benefitted less from their parents' participation in treatment. Fortunately, there is also evidence that early intervention with such high callous–unemotional children holds the promise of restoring their developmental progress, when using a multimodal treatment package with a high level of parental involvement, focused on the creation of a warm supportive parent–child relationship, which facilitates emotional learning. As is so often the case in medicine, the earlier we intervene, the greater the chances to arrest negative development and outcomes.

Our review of existing medication and other biological interventions shows very little progress in the past 5 to 10 years. There are few novel compounds; we still have no specific indication for the treatment of aggression, as for instance exists for pain or fever. Without such indication we cannot expect to see a large increase in funding of medication trials. At best, we have some good reports of medication efficacy in the context of other diagnoses, such as ADHD. However, while there is growing awareness on how medications can be useful in this difficult population, a systematic and sophisticated understanding of how exactly to proceed is under discussion and construction. At best, the current studies are characterized as promissory notes, without many gold standard randomized double blind placebo controlled trials in evidence. This is disappointing and we suggest not reflective of the true potential of psychopharmacology to significantly contribute to the therapeutics of DBDs.

With regard to social interventions, Multisystemic Therapy is backed by a large body of data and international contributions. This modality aims at helping the most severe forms of DBDs in the adolescent age range, especially a much-needed addition to our armamentarium. These studies are impressive, and their replication in different countries on different continents is encouraging. However, many of these studies are somewhat dismissive of concurrent medication treatment, which is usually delivered in an ad hoc fashion, very often driven by emergencies. The most impressive aspect of these studies is the demonstration that careful manualization of interventions can lead to good outcomes in some of the most disturbed and morbid populations.

Again, on the positive side, we have reached a stage of empirical knowledge allowing us to develop more sophisticated multimodal intervention studies, comparing, for example, medication and behavioral treatments, as well as combinations of these different modalities. Without this information, the clinician is still in a great predicament: When does he or she use one versus the other; when are combinations indicated? Is the selection of treatment method driven by acuity, chronicity, phenotype of symptom, setting for the intervention? All of these questions remain unanswered at this point. Without this knowledge, it is extremely difficult to deliver precision medical care. Too many of the treatment studies of, for example, medication treatment are silent concerning the concurrent behavioral or institutional treatments that in all likelihood have some treatment effects. By the same token, many of the studies of behavioral interventions, especially those reporting results in highly compromised populations, say little about medication use. We have not progressed too far from the recommendations issued by the Stanford/Howard Workgroup on Juvenile Impulsivity and Aggression, sponsored in part by the American Academy of Child & Adolescent Psychiatry and chaired by one of us (HS) in 2006. The group developed a consensus that several medications showed promise in the treatment of maladaptive aggression, such as atypical antipsychotics, divalproex sodium, lithium, and for youth with conduct problems and ADHD, stimulant medications. But there is only very little additional empirical evidence to strengthen this recommendation, especially if one only considers studies that use the DBD diagnoses as the primary inclusion criterion. There are newer studies, but most of them report on the treatment of antisocial behavior and aggression in the context of other primary diagnoses (such as ADHD). Fortunately, we have developed an advanced methodological tool that will permit us to acquire much-needed information. The use of a sequential multiple assignment randomized trial (SMART; Armirall, Nahum-Shani, Sherwood, & Murphy, 2014) will hopefully be applied in many future research studies and answer some of the questions we have raised in the treatment chapter.

The other hope is that by increasingly crisp and specific subtypification of DBDs there will be greater precision in matching symptom to treatment. We also have to remain cautious: while for instance callous–unemotional traits have shown some promise in subtyping DBDs in a way that ultimately will prove helpful, we still need to be aware of the limits inherent in this construct. The Kolko and Pardini (2010) study demonstrates this for DBDs in the context of ADHD: callous–unemotional traits did not bear any discernible relation to outcomes three years posttreatment. In addition to inducing some skepticism in the clinical arena, such findings also have potential implications for the legal status of the patient and the managing forensic entities. The world of the law and criminology perpetually seeks predictors of dangerousness, risk for relapse, and so on. Callous–unemotional traits are often thought to be helpful in this regard. But we have to keep in mind that the more recent meta-analyses (e.g. Hawes, Price, & Dadds, 2014) showed that while callous–unemotional traits are, in fact, associated with poorer treatment outcomes, certain parent training interventions can attenuate callous–unemotional traits, especially if applied early in the course of illness. Callous–unemotional does not seem synonymous with permanently incorrigible.

There are still many unanswered questions regarding the best treatment of DBDs in males versus females. Throughout the literature, it is evident that girls and boys differ in their symptomatology, diagnostic profiles, and baseline characteristics, which moderate and mediate treatment. There continues to be a great need for large-scale studies of differential treatment outcomes in the two genders.

Finally, we also need treatment studies which investigate neurobiological correlates and predictors of treatment effects. Stadler and colleagues (2008) provide a model study for this line of investigation, which is ongoing and is yielding several interesting early results. Examining the efficacy of a comprehensive skills training program for female adolescents with ODD and CD on emotion regulation both on a behavioral and a neurobiological level pre–post to intervention compared to treatment as usual, the group was better able to define bottom-up (biology influences and changes psychology and social causal loops) or top-down effects (psychology or social interventions have effects on biology).

A good summary of the status of the treatment literature of DBDs is that therapeutic nihilism is currently not valid. Several meta-analyses support at least significant modest effects of psychosocial interventions on antisocial behavior. We are convinced that psychosocial intervention effectiveness could be even increased, if we aim to better tailor interventions to various aggression phenotypes. A similar conclusion can probably also be applied to biological treatments. The task is to develop criteria and then apply precision health care to DBDs. The other major conclusion from the existing data is that the closer we keep studies in the real world to studies in nonclinical, experimental settings by insisting on a high level of protocol fidelity and training and supervision of the staff involved in real-world clinical settings, the greater the chances that we can obtain much improved outcomes. The protocols and structures emerging from tightly controlled clinical trials can lead to considerable progress in the clinical world of DBDs, similar to what has been shown to be the case in the treatment of ADHD, when treatment as usual and research protocols were compared.

Such expectations also should be extended to juvenile justice settings where it all too often is the case that, at best, ineffective and, at worst, injurious protocols are being applied without any empirical evidence that patients benefit. Good examples are wilderness programs without follow-up or the Scared Straight programs involving juveniles' visits to imprisoned adults. Similar concerns can be raised about the extensive and untargeted use of potentially harmful medications throughout juvenile justice and residential treatment settings, as well as settings involving youth in foster care. This issue has been raised quite forcefully in the past decade and justifiably so.

These persistent misapplications of well-meaning interventions also show that there is a great gap in disseminating the best and latest findings from the literature on DBDs to the relevant clinics, residential settings, and juvenile justice facilities and their staff. As we discussed in chapter 6 on forensics, we need to create innovative pathways and programs for such educational interventions. In the absence of such changes, we can expect that one of the main problems in staffing facilities treating youths with DBDs will persist: staff burn out, resulting in either inappropriate staff behavior or high staff turnover. One such good example of how to address some of these issues is the use of motivational interviewing, which has been manualized and tested. Results have been positive, as Miller and Rollnik (2012) have shown. In addition, the UK-based NICE network has developed specific guidelines for use in staff training.

The good news is that our knowledge regarding treatment of DBDs has expanded enormously in the past 5 to 10 years. The bad news is that with the acquisition of such a broad database we now know, definitively, that in treating DBDs there is no one approach that fits all.

In chapter 6, "Forensic Implications in Disruptive Behavior Disorders," we bring together the current knowledge of DBDs and the legal standards and landmark legal cases that influence medical practice for patients with DBDs. In a certain way, DBDs can be looked as "medical speak" for juvenile crime and delinquency. We examined the factors that have influenced the confluence of psychiatric medicine and juvenile justice. We also looked at the mutual benefits and conflicts that inevitably arise when these two systems (medicine and the law) begin to assume joint responsibility in rehabilitating and treating a group of very complex patients. Finally, we explored the ways that our criminal justice system may be forced to adapt in the years to come as our knowledge base of DBDs and their successful rehabilitation increases.

Basically, criminology approaches crime and the criminal or delinquent from a sociological/cultural perspective. From such a perspective, delinquents are seen as being part of a subculture that needs to be changed. Criminological "treatment" approaches to crime and delinquency center on safety, security, assessment of risk, retribution, and punishment. They focus much less on rehabilitation, re-education, or medical treatment. By contrast, the medical perspective is heavily individualistic. A person who may have committed crimes is a patient; he or she suffers a disorder. That person is granted the protection of the sick role—up to a point. The issues of free will and culpability require reexamination and potential recalibration, as our knowledge from neuroscience and empirical studies regarding the causes and manifestations of DBDs expands. Determinism, which is the subject—rightfully—of a vigorous debate in the neurosciences, stands in sharp contrast to the legal assumption that as long as a person is mentally competent to stand trial for a crime and meets a jurisdictional legal standard for sanity at the time of said crime, he or she is in principle capable to be guilty. However, recent findings from medicine and neuroscience may essentially force a reexamination from the point of view of an empirical, evidence-based biology, psychology, and sociology in the coming years. Are youth who have committed serious crimes amoral criminals, or are they patients? Do such youth need "treatment" potentially consisting of medication, psychotherapy, remedial education, and/or neurofeedback? Or, on the contrary, do they need to spend time in juvenile detention and/or prisons pondering the consequences of their decisions? Is our role to protect society from such persons, or can help and compassion stop them from committing similar crimes in the future?

The answers to these questions should be driven by a few important considerations. First, DBDs and externalizing disorders, as a matter of clinical fact, very often need containment and behavioral control that is not available in psychiatric settings, especially when such containment is needed over extended periods of time. Justice settings with their focus on safety, security, and control are much better equipped to handle this, while at the same time fulfilling society's demands that the perpetrators of severe crime be punished. Second, given that a large portion of delinquents are highly psychiatrically morbid and comorbid, we need to apply the available tools of modern medicine to the treatment of these youngsters. We are still faced with the problem of having psychiatrically extremely morbid patients in justice system institutions that are frequently not well equipped to handle such complicated psychiatric cases. Although we cannot—for safety and security reasons—completely replicate the structures of sophisticated intensivist settings in medicine in justice settings, we should be able to provide state-of-the-art care in integrated services stratified through the justice facilities. Following an exhaustive and detailed assessment of the California Youth Authority, we are better able to conceptualize the need of the youths in that system and propose institutional changes holding great promise for improved outcomes. Such changes—in net effect—would require the development of specialized institutional clinics (internalizing, externalizing, rare and unusual, mild to moderate substance use, moderate to severe substance use) clustering the most commonly found psychopathologies into populations treated by a team of experts in the respective clusters. We have generated strong data support from a very large-scale and representative study of the California Youth Authority that proposes a way of streamlining services in this particular way, which maximizes existing resources within the justice system. Such a reorganization holds great promise for improved outcomes while being optimally efficient.

In addition, we have learned a great deal from medical and neuroscientific data regarding the outpatient and postinstitutional management of delinquent youth. We have learned that factors of paramount importance to facilitating youths' rehabilitation and reintegration into the community include, but are not limited to, the following: preserving access to mental health services by designing step-down and diversion programs supervised by special courts, such as drug and mental health; ceasing to commit youths with relatively minor crimes immediately to long-term incarceration settings; keeping family contacts intact before, during and after a criminological treatment phase. These changes ultimately should translate into reduced recidivism.

The mental health practitioner interested in consulting and interacting with the world of the law needs to be prepared to encounter some challenges and obstacles. The intensified infusion of medical and neuroscientific facts into the world of the law and criminology often brings unexpected fallout that runs counter to our role as practitioners of medicine. The vignette chronicling the care of a young man named Jay is a good illustration of the sort of challenged posted when providing care in criminal and/or juvenile justice settings. Mental health professionals will need to navigate the inevitable conflicts that often arise between themselves and institutional guidelines in a collegial and professional manner in order to preserve our autonomy and efficacy and provide the best care possible.

Given the influx of new information about DBDs, we are now in a much better position to tackle one of the most important theoretical issues: the redefinition of standards of culpability. Influencing the law in this regard will be a tough task, especially when faced with all the problematic aspects of our current DBD labels. In their present form, they will not lead to any consideration by the law to exculpate perpetrators. For example, the mitigating influence of mental illness (irresistible impulse defense) on criminal culpability was significantly reduced following John Hinckley Jr.'s attempted assassination of President Ronald Reagan.

Under some circumstances, juvenile courts will pose questions like "What implications does this (DBD) diagnosis have for the future of this defendant? How will treatment(s) work to ascertain his/her future risk for reoffending?" Given what we currently know, the DBD labels are not helpful in answering either of these questions. But this may be a more reachable goal in the near future. It may also serve as an intermediary step to an ultimate answer regarding culpability. For now, the DBD labels are simply not good enough to surpass the aid forensic psychiatry receives from those arguments related to developmental immaturity. DBD diagnoses in and of themselves do not add much to such discussions.

It is fair to say that—as noted in almost all of the chapters—much work still needs to be done in the forensics area. We have indeed come a long way in gaining the respect and attention of our colleagues in the world of law and criminology. This has happened by becoming more independent from these worlds but not separated from them. Being ready to step in and help with the most difficult clinical situations one can imagine has worked in our favor, judging by the rapid increase of requests for consultation to all kinds of cases from lawyers, judges, and directors of county and state facilities. However, such requests by far exceed our capacity to respond. This is yet another rewarding and stimulating career path that will require new trainees in forensic psychiatry and much applied research and understanding of basic research for many decades to come. This appears to be an area of almost guaranteed "job security" for empathic and inspired young clinicians for the foreseeable future. We hope to have provided a significant basis for a decision to join us and help all of us involved in doing what we do best: bring hope and healing to those who suffer in the most unimaginable and complicated way.

The following are some resources readers can consult for further information.

American Academy of Child & Adolescent Psychiatry: "The mission of AACAP is to promote the healthy development of children, adolescents, and families through advocacy, education, and research, and to meet the professional needs of child and adolescent psychiatrists throughout their careers."

http://www.aacap.org/AACAP/About_AACAP/Home.aspx

American Academy of Pediatrics: "The mission of the American Academy of Pediatrics is to attain optimal physical, mental, and social health and well-being for all infants, children, adolescents and young adults."

https://www.aap.org/en-us/Pages/Default.aspx

Centers for Disease Control and Prevention: "[the] CDC works 24/7 to protect America from health, safety and security threats, both foreign and in the U.S."

http://www.cdc.gov/about/organization/mission.htm

The National Institute for Health and Care Excellence: "provides national guidance and advice to improve health and social care."

https://www.nice.org.uk/about

National Institute of Justice: the research, development, and evaluation agency of the US Department of Justice. Its mission focuses on the application of science to further understanding within the field of crime and justice.

https://www.nij.gov/Pages/welcome.aspx

Oregon Social Learning Center: A nonprofit research center that focuses on effects of social and psychological processes on individuals and their families. Information gleaned from this research is translated and applied to their everyday life of individuals and their families, extending to their communities.

http://www.oslc.org

References

Almirall, D., Nahum-Shani, I., Sherwood, N. E., & Murphy, S. A. (2014). Introduction to SMART designs for the development of adaptive interventions: With application to weight loss research. *Translational Behavioral Medicine, 4*(3), 260–274.

Epstein, R. A., Fonnesbeck, C., Potter, S., Rizzone, K. H., & McPheeters, M. (2015). Psychosocial interventions for child disruptive behaviors: A meta-analysis. *Pediatrics, 136*(5), 2015–2577.

Hawes, D. J., Price, M. J., & Dadds, M. R. (2014). Callous-unemotional traits and the treatment of conduct problems in childhood and adolescence: A comprehensive review. *Clinical Child and Family Psychology Review, 17*(3), 248–267.

Kolko, D. J., & Pardini, D. A. (2010). ODD dimensions, ADHD, and callous–unemotional traits as predictors of treatment response in children with disruptive behavior disorders. *Journal of Abnormal Psychology, 119*(4), 713–725.

Miller, W. R., & Rollnick, S. (2012). *Motivational interviewing: Helping people change.* New York: Guilford Press.

Stadler, C., Grasmann, D., Fegert, J. M., Holtmann, M., Poustka, F., & Schmeck, K. (2008). Heart rate and treatment effect in children with disruptive behavior disorders. *Child Psychiatry and Human Development, 39*(3), 299–309.

Index

Page references for figures are indicated by *f,* for tables by *t,* and for boxes by *b.*